Symmetry
Enhanced Health
And Performance

Relieve Pain

and

Optimize Physical Motion

New Techniques To Maximize
Comfort and Control Over Your Body

Richard R. Johnson
Patrick R. Mummy

Quantum Media

Symmetry, Enhanced Health and Performance

Other Titles and Future Projects by Richard R. Johnson:
Find Anyone Right Now
Sales 2000
The Circles of Balance
Instant Financial Survival
The Interactive Guide To Health & Ideal Weight
Forms Galore
Mastering The Internet
The Interactive Guide To Patents

Copyright 1999 by Quantum Media, Inc.

Printed in the United States Of America

Publication Data:

Symmetry / Richard R. Johnson,
Patrick R. Mummy

ISBN 1-893477-01-0
1. Health
2. Exercise

Published by Quantum Media
1340 Enterprise Drive
Romeoville, IL 60446

http://www.cdpublisher.com

**Increased Energy, Pain Relief, Enhanced Performance
and a Greater Sense of Well-Being are the Results
of Applying Symmetry to Your Life.**

Throughout my life, I have attempted to learn as much as possible about enhancing and promoting my overall health and physical performance. I've seen and experienced countless programs and systems all promoting health and improved fitness. Virtually all of the programs and techniques had an obvious downside, or were too difficult to maintain for the period of time required for positive results. The bottom line is, they just didn't work for me. Then I found Symmetry.

The concepts and techniques taught in Symmetry are quite basic, and in their simplicity, resides incredible power and exceptional results. Symmetry makes sense. The payoff can be almost instant and the techniques are practical for an entire lifetime. During my first go-around with the information, I found that the approach felt very comfortable and realistic. The second go-around, I began to truly understand the power of Symmetry's postural therapy.

The first thing I noticed was that I felt more comfortable after eating. Then my swimming stroke got stronger and more consistent. Soon, the occasional weakness and pain in my right knee from an old football injury, subsided. Virtually every aspect of my physical performance has been enhanced and improved as a result of applying the processes taught in Symmetry. I have enjoyed it so much that I have written a book and CD-ROM about it . What more can I say?

Enjoy....
        Richard R. Johnson

Thanks from Patrick R. Mummy...

So many people have been instrumental in the successful completion of this project. I regret that I am not able to thank each and everyone of you personally.

I would like to take this opportunity to name a few special people. First and foremost my wife Lauren Jacobsen Mummy, without whose love and support, this would not have been possible. Sincere thanks also to all of the dedicated and passionate Symmetry folk, in particular, Amanda Jacobsen and Anna-Maja Dahlgren, whose commitment and constant pursuit of excellence keeps this company progressing to greater heights. Thanks to all the wonderful and talented people at Quantum Media.

Thanks to our clients, without whom we would not have a purpose and mission in life. Special thanks to Chris Rodahaffer for taking the risk. Thanks to Michael Mack, Tom Vardell, Pat Jeane, Dr. Mark Kalina, Eric Faulk, Shawn Michaels, KUSI News and Charles Pelletier for their endorsement and faith in us. Heartfelt thanks to Ivor and Joan Jacobsen for their unconditional love, endless generosity, and unwavering support.

Thanks from Richard R. Johnson...

My deepest appreciation goes out to Rob and the "R.D. Team," Patrick and Lauren Mummy, Tom Palmer, Chris Rodahaffer, Pat Sayor, Brittin Taylor, Carole Pecora, Greg Baumann and my wife Cindy, for her patience and understanding for my hours at the office.

NOTE: Don't Forget to Use The CD-ROM...

Section 1. The Basics and General Overview

Section 2. Introduction to Body Types in Exercises

Section 3. The Exercises Shown Alphabetically

Appendix A

Appendix B

This book was developed and produced as a companion to the CD-ROM program included. Many sections of the book were first written as script outlines for the audio narrations on the CD-ROM. In order to maintain continuity and consistent language between the CD-ROM and the book, the writing style utilized within the book is more narrative and relaxed than conventional modern English writing styles.

This program offers techniques that may not be appropriate for everyone. We strongly advise that all indivduals seek the councel of their own personal medical doctor before engaging in any personal health related exercise program.

Neither the authors or Quantum Media, Inc. shall be liable or responsible regarding any loss, injury or damage caused or alleged to be caused directly or indirectly by the information contained in this book or the utilization of the CD-ROM software program contained herein. It is further understood that the authors are not medical doctors and are not engaged in the process of rendering medical advice or other professional medical services.

Who could get the most out of this program?

At this point, that is indeed the most relevant question. The answer is almost anyone, but there is some qualification required here. People who experience chronic pain, especially those whose pain was caused by an injury, are perfectly suited for this. Athletes of all types should understand and utilize the underlying principles for greater endurance and performance. People who feel that age is becoming a factor in their lives would do well to master the techniques taught here. It may seem as though anyone in any condition would be suited for this program, but that is not necessarily the case.

The concepts in postural therapy take for granted that the individuals learning the techniques have a standard baseline of physical ability. It is important to understand that the methods utilized in this program require a minimum level of mobility. Even people who are in a condition requiring the use of a wheelchair and are otherwise quite healthy, may find quite a few useful bits of information and techniques here.

Notwithstanding individuals who are not as fortunate as those with a realistic potential of great health in motion, all others will find the information contained in this program to be useful and beneficial. The techniques and concepts are designed to be used and appreciated by people who want to improve their health, strength, energy, endurance, comfort, reaction time and sleep. Yes, we did mention sleep, because optimal postural alignment benefits sleep patterns as well. If there are specific attributes of good health that we have overlooked, we apologize — because we hope to improve those as well. We estimate that virtually every aspect related to the improvement of health can be intertwined with the subject of postural therapy.

Anything that's done to improve health will be negated to some degree if posture is overlooked as part of their health improvement program. Muscles, bones, nerves, tendons, circulation, respiration and internal organs all benefit from postural alignment.
We do not profess that proper posture is the end all and be all to good health, but it may well be the most greatly overlooked facet of human health. We often hear about the quality of air, or the quality of water, and certainly the quality of food. All of these can

factor greatly into the health and well-being of an individual. Also, these particular requirements or necessities of health have products and services tied to them. In other words, promoters of such products and services all have something to sell. When we talk about postural alignment, there isn't a lot to sell with regard to products and services. In its purest form, it is information and techniques which, after obtained, are free for the taking to be enjoyed by everyone. Almost everything you need to know and will learn about this subject can be practiced with typical household items such as a belt, a footstool, a chair, and a wall.

Most of us live lives that could be improved with postural therapy. Very simply put, the body works better when its parts are lined up and positioned as they were designed. It is realistic to assume that most peoples bodies need some work and attention. That is a very politically correct way of saying that we all have some physical problems. Attention is the keyword here. The problem is that many people are not paying attention to the messages that their bodies are sending. But there is one message that almost no one can ignore.

Quite often the message that the body sends the loudest is pain. Make no mistake, pain is a message. Pain tells you what's wrong and even offers suggestions on how to fix it. The problem is that your body typically sends a quick-fix message. For example, if you sprain your left ankle, your body tells you to take pressure off of the left side and shift it over to the right. This is a quick fix, also considered a reaction, and is instinctive. Any animal and even insects know that when one leg is injured, they need to compensate with the others.

It is this basic instinct to compensate that can be the start of many physical ailments to come. In time, one body part learns to compensate for another and soon some muscles atrophy while others grow and strengthen. During the healing process, one of the main considerations is comfort, because naturally people want to be comfortable and pain free. They will do whatever is necessary to obtain that position, but eventually it could lead to more pain than they bargained for.

Of course, there is the more popular path to postural malady, which is good old- fashioned habits. Or more to the point, bad habits. If all of us were to collect a quarter for every time we heard, "sit up straight, stand up straight or quit slouching," while growing up, we'd have a nice nest egg. Many will argue that habits are hard to break, and if this program is about breaking habits or a major change in lifestyle, then they will have no part of it. It's perfectly understandable that people are tired of being preached to, and we do not want to preach to anyone. But believe it or not, there are some techniques that when utilized correctly can actually retrain the body to hold itself and move better. Surprisingly, some of these techniques can have very speedy results and often have people on the way to improvement in just one session. That subject is essentially the driving concept and basis for this program and we hope you enjoy it as much as we do living it.

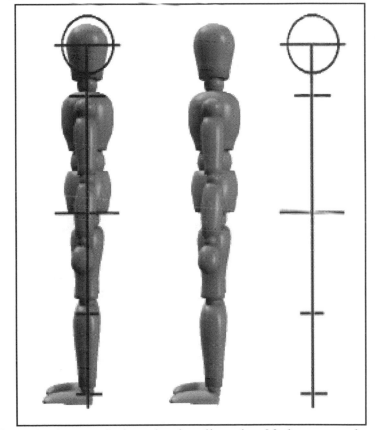

Your body was designed to be aligned at 90 degree angles.

How Did I Get Here?

You may be wondering how you got to the point where you felt the necessity of a new direction in managing your pain or improving your dynamics of motion. Or maybe your situation might not be directly related to pain, but more related to a condition that's bothersome or problematic. Perhaps you're looking for a new way to add motion dynamics to your lifestyle or sport. Regardless of your situation or desire, you have found yourself in a position that requires a remedy or improvement. If you have a problem, you will learn how to fix it, and you will also learn techniques and methods to prevent its return. But for now let's take a look at your lifestyle — a few examples — and try to get a handle on what has motivated you to improve, heal or advance.

Your problem may not technically be a problem at all, rather it may be a condition, or circumstance that you would like to see changed or improved. Many people do not like to consider their circumstance as problematic, sensing that problems are troublesome or negative. When we refer to problems, we're actually considering the term as it relates to a challenge or desire for change. In consideration of your situation, it is important to relate to the positive aspects of your direction and desire. Regardless of why you've chosen to seek out a new means to greater health, your action of contemplating a new, positive direction is a big plus and should be applauded.

First of all, what kind of person are you? How's that for a loaded question? What we're looking for here is a baseline, or some guide that you can use to measure how you fit in. The objective here is to create a baseline for comparative purposes, because without a measurable outline, there can be no basis for performance or growth.

Can you run a marathon? Can you walk a marathon? Are you strong? Can you lift a lot of weight for your size? Can you go all day without getting tired? Has a doctor told you that you are in great shape? Has a health professional told you that you need some level of improvement?

As you can surmise at this point, there is no end to the number of questions one can ask regarding one's state of health. Actually, it's a very difficult task to quantify because there are so many variables and baselines. A doctor might consider your condition and health to be excellent, and yet you may fail miserably at a triathlon qualification. Another aspect of your health and conditioning that needs to be considered is your aerobic conditioning. You might statistically have the perfect balance of weight for your height and the ideal body fat count. You might also have excellent vital statistics such as: blood pressure, pulse rate and reflexes. Now you can see why it is so difficult to gauge and quantify someone's health. Thankfully, the measure of ideal postural health is readily detectable by anyone with a little training. Still, for your purposes as a guide, place yourself where you think you fit in on the health-in-motion ladder.

Everybody has a position on the ladder of health in motion. People on the bottom of the ladder have a serious condition which prevents, or seriously inhibits, unassisted mobility. People on the bottom of the health-in-motion ladder cannot get around on their own power. That is not to say that they are unhealthy, because their health in general may be just fine, but if their motion is severely limited, then we must consider the condition to be serious.

The last thing we want to do is to seem cruel or cold-hearted with a basis or definition. In reality, if you want to have any realistic chance at changing your health situation, you must have an idea of where you stand in relation to others. Someone at the bottom of the health ladder needs help with day to day living and movement. This is a person who cannot get up and walk around on their own. They have trouble eating on their own, and for all practical purposes, require a full-time nurse or medical assistant to sustain life. So now you have an idea of what the bottom of the health-in-motion ladder is regarding your position on it.

With a good idea of where you might fall on the health-in-motion ladder, what do you suppose the attributes would be for someone placed at the top? At this point, you don't have the benefit of understanding what ideal postural alignment is, and that makes this concept particularly interesting. For our purposes, someone at the top of the ladder would have the abilities and fitness attributes of an Olympic gymnast. Their body would be upright with straight shoulders, lean body mass, excellent strength, incredible agility, and a marathon runner's endurance. Naturally, there aren't dozens of other considerations, but bear in mind that we are shooting for an ideal here, and not a specific profile regarding all aspects of health.

Here are a few questions that you can answer with a rating number from 1-5. After all the questions have been answered, add up your score, then compare your score with our baseline. Remember, you are the one who is standardizing your physical condition. A low score will give you a place to start from with lots of room for improvement. A high score might indicate one of two things: one, you were not completely honest with yourself on the scoring; or two, although you may be in excellent condition, your performance level may have peaked, indicating improvement may be needed in other areas as well.

Part 1 Flexibility
1. Touch toes with fingers and knees locked — standing position
2. Touch toes with fingers and knees locked — seated position
3. Body bridge — palms and feet flat on floor, stomach arched up
4. Touch fingers, one arm back over shoulder, other arm back, point ing up.
5. Seated on floor — V-sit, Chinese splits

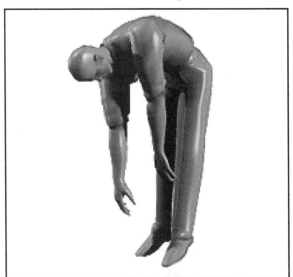

Obviously some movements and exercises will be harder if not virtually impossible for some people to do. Don't let it bother you, just do the best you can, see page 8 chart.

Part 2 Strength
1. Push-ups
2. Pull-ups
3. Squats
4. Sit-ups

Part 3 Endurance
1. Jogging
2. Running
3. Jumping Jacks

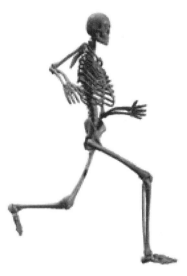

Most of us have had the opportunity of watching people around us move up and down on a ladder of health. I have seen individuals that I considered to be somewhere in the middle of the ladder move to the top and to the bottom within a year's time.

In all fairness, most of us have seen professional athletes who might be considered at the top of the ladder move to the bottom during the course of a game. There they are in all their glory running for a touchdown, when all of a sudden someone comes in hard from the side and hits them right at the knees. The crowd is silenced, the team is stunned, the coach bows his head, hoping and praying that it's not the worst. After taking the hit, the player lies still, maybe a little bit in shock, but knowing that lying still is the best thing he can do. He's not sure if he's hurt, but oddly he checks out the leg that wasn't hit first. Then he flexes his muscle slightly, and stretches a little bit. This gives him a quick reminder of what a healthy leg should feel like. Now with some anticipation, he flexes the leg that took the hit. "A little numb," he thinks, "but no pain and that's a good sign." Now he goes for the stretch: he moves a little and then tries to move a little more. "Not bad," he thinks. "Feels about like the other leg. I think I can get up."

At about the same moment, he decides to get up by himself, surrounded by teammates and the team doctor. They ask him how he feels, he shakes his head and tells them, "I think I'm okay." Just the same, for the sake of precaution, the team doctor and one of the players each grab a shoulder and help him up.

Part 1 Flexibility

1. Touch toes standing

☐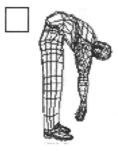

2. Touch toes seated on floor

☐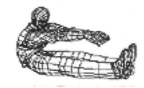

4. Touch fingers over shoulder reach

☐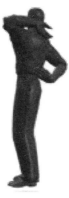

3. Body bridge

☐

5. Seated on floor — V-sit, Chinese splits

☐

Part 2 Strength

1. Push-ups	
2. Pull-ups	
3. Squats	
4. Sit-ups	

Part 3 Endurance

1. Jogging	
2. Running	
3. Jumping Jacks	

INSTRUCTIONS

There are 12 boxes to fill in rating 1-5.
A total score of 12 is the lowest. 60 is the highest you can go.
Average score is 30.

"How's that feel?" the team doctor asks.

"Not bad," responds our hero.

The coach looks on from afar, almost as though he can hear every word. By gestures alone, he knows exactly what's going on and the worst part is that there is nothing he can do about it.

"How about trying to put a little weight on that," says the team doctor.

"I thought I was," says the player.

"No, we've been holding you up the whole time. You might be in a little shock. I want you to take it real easy and real slow — let's see if your leg will take the pressure," replies the doctor.

The player takes a look at the coach, the coach looks back, and then puts his head down. At this point, he knows that this is serious even before the player. The player tries to put some weight on his leg and finds out what the coach already knew: the leg is badly injured.
That is a typical example of someone who was at the top of the health-in-motion ladder one minute, and at the very next was near the bottom.

Let's go back for a moment and take a look at how we define health. Realizing that the concept of health as an end in itself is quite subjective, we need to place some parameters on the subject. Certainly, bedridden hospital patients are considered to be in a serious situation. Obviously, each situation is different: some may be temporary, others may be terminal. Remember, for our purposes here, anyone that requires the assistance of someone else to move about or sustain themselves will be defined as surviving at the bottom of the ladder. This certainly does not mean that they are any less of a person in any regard — it simply gives an idea of where they stand on the health in motion ladder.

Pain — The Four-Letter Word

Pain is a four-letter word and can be one of the most frustrating aspects of human life. Often pain is habitual and potentially inherited. Pain can be chronic from the standpoint of day-to-day living such as: sleeping patterns, sitting postures, daily work routines, or restrictive clothing and shoes. Perhaps walking styles, standing postures, the way one moves in a shower, and literally hundreds of other possibilities are potential factors.

Each of us has several conditions in and around all facets of daily living, and physical attributes which lead to pain. These conditions are called perpetuating factors. Perpetuating factors of pain are typically handled with quick fixes such as drugs, shoe lifts and ergonomic furniture. Billions and billions of dollars are poured into markets every year due to catchy advertising and simple ignorance of the factors that perpetuate pain. If you have a headache, drugs are the typical quick fix, and in this case the drugs are part of the perpetuating factor. An example of this concept would be someone who sits incorrectly for most of the day and causes muscles to contract in the back or neck, which eventually leads to a headache. Let's add up the perpetuating factors:

First, you have the condition or situation which leads to the sitting all day. In most cases, that situation will be work and there may not be anything you can do to change the work, but you might be able to change how you work.

Second, you must consider the position you're sitting in and why you are sitting in that position. Is it because it's more comfortable, or because it's painful to sit in other positions? After a short period of time, your actions become habits and, of course, habits are hard to break.

Third, there is the quick-fix habit of taking a pain-relieving drug when the pain starts. There's nothing wrong with wanting pain to go away, but if you take a pain reliever and continue doing something that's causing the pain, then you simply perpetuate the condition.

Often the medical community and other health practitioners offer equipment, furniture and various devices and methods to help alleviate pain. The medical community will focus on the specific symptoms of the pain and usually attempt to treat the symptoms. Health practitioners and therapists often look for the causes of symptoms and attempt to treat those. There are hundreds, if not thousands of pieces of equipment and health-related paraphernalia aimed at quickly treating pain. People want their pain to go away so badly that they will turn to anything to find relief. The faster the better, and quite often the more bizarre, the faster customers will line up for a try at the latest, greatest, fastest pain reliever of all time. With the predictability of daybreak, their pain returns, although people will often say that it worked for a little while, or relieved their pain to some degree just to save face. All the while, the permanent relief of pain is right in front of you — literally in a mirror just waiting to be diagnosed and evaluated. The first step to relieving your pain starts with an honest self-evaluation.

At some point, you will learn to be a pain detective looking for all types of causes for your pain. You will no doubt learn several new techniques while becoming a pain detective, such as noticing how other people go about the motions involved in their daily lives. You may observe someone's sitting posture and think to yourself, "That can't be good for their back."

One of the best methods of learning to gauge your pain is to carry along a recorder or notebook. When you find yourself in a position that causes pain from some part of your body, make note of the situation so you can make the proper changes in the future. Remember, you can learn new techniques for fixing your pain, but if you keep doing the same things over and over, you'll find yourself back in the same condition of habitual pain.

Habits form quickly with repetition, and nothing creates repetition like a daily routine and schedule. You may get up for work, shower and go out for the paper at the same time everyday. Then you find yourself at work standing in the same places and sitting in the same positions day in and day out. One trick in dealing with pain is to discover **methods of relief. Methods of relief** are any motions or changes in physical position that you do in order to relieve an ache or pain. It might be as simple as leaning forward at your desk, or it might be as complicated as getting up and walking over to the water cooler or coffee room. As a matter of habit, people often find themselves in positions that will quickly create a pain, but since the relief method is habitual, they might not even consciously notice that they had the pain in the first place. This is why it's so important to take notice of methods of relief so you can record what positions or activities caused the pain in the first place.

Now let's have a look at how you may have found yourself requiring a remedy for your condition. Do you consider yourself a creature of habit? Do you get up at the same time everyday? Is your routine virtually unvaried on a daily basis? What about the furniture in your life? Do you sit in the same chair at the same time every day? Do you sleep in the same position every night? Do you remember to turn your mattress and rotate it every two weeks? That seems like a tall order, but it really can help your back and the life of your mattress. I'm sure you get the idea here: if you find yourself doing the same things every day and every night at virtually the same times, and you experience similar pains on a regular basis, then it's time for a change in routine.

Let's start with how you wake up and get out of bed in the morning. One very useful technique in avoiding pain and injury is to not jump out of bed as soon as you wake up. Consider this from a physiological point of view: one of the first things you need to do when you awaken is to get your respiratory system up to speed. If you're the average person, you breathe easily, that is, without too much effort throughout the night. As a result, your heart rate is down and your respiratory rate is also less burdened than during your day-to-day activities. If you jump out of bed the second you wake up, you're asking your body to jump into overdrive before you get your engine started. Take a little time to wake up in the morning — it's okay to stretch a little bit and get your eyes focused before you plunge into your day. Many people don't consider how well their body works when it's replenished with oxygen. When you consciously take the time for a few deep breaths, your heart rate will go up and your body will prepare itself for action. Would you ever consider giving someone directions for a task when you felt they might not be prepared for it physically? Then why put yourself directly into harm's way by rushing into action when your body isn't ready?

Now that we have your wake-up routine in question and perhaps under some new scrutiny, let's move on to what typically happens next. Or more to the point, what should happen next. Assuming that you've taken a moment for a deep breath or two and allowed your eyes to focus, consider what should be your next move. How about a little stretching? We're not talking about a full routine requiring a new time commitment, but rather quite simply, a little stretching. Considering actual time, we're talking about less than a minute to move most of your major parts. A lot of people find themselves injured or in pain just moments after they get out of bed. Unknowingly, they may have slept in an unusual position throughout the night, which may have caused some shortening of muscle tissue, or stiffness in the joints. If you jump out of bed after such an evening, you may injure yourself. This makes perfect sense when you think about it, because you have no idea what positions you have been sleeping in throughout the night, and therefore cannot possibly be prepared for every potential body movement the following morning. So slow down just a little, and that will help you prepare yourself for whatever comes next in your daily routine.

Honest Performance Evaluation

This program falls under the "self-help" category in book stores and catalogs. That's not to say that this program could not be used with groups or teams, but in actuality it's marketed for individual use. The problem with self-help products is that the individuals who buy them are not always honest with their personal evaluations, which often are required with a program. This program also falls into the health and medical categories in bookstores and catalogs. One concept regarding medical evaluations which simply never works is a lack of honesty. You must be completely honest with yourself regarding medical evaluations. If it hurts, say it hurts. If you can't do something, don't say you can. You get the idea — honesty is the best policy when it comes to a performance evaluation.

The idea of a performance evaluation is centered around the physical activities that you do the most. Let's say that you like to play basketball, and the last time you played basketball you were not satisfied with your performance. Or maybe you like to go out dancing and the next day you feel stiff and sore. I am certain you're beginning to get the idea — whatever it is you do in motion, whether it be a sport or hobby, sometimes you feel great about it and other times you feel disappointed. Our goal is to get you to feel better about your performance in motion. As we mentioned before, we are also concerned with other aspects of your health such as: your respiratory system, circulatory system and so on. Aside from your vitals, we are looking to help you gauge your personal performance. What's good, what's bad, are there noticeable improvements or have things gone downhill?

Here are some factors to consider that will help you formulate an honest performance evaluation:

1. The three activities in motion that you do the most
2. The dates when you first started each of these activities.
3. Use of the following chart for a performance/improvement.

Make 3 copies of the of the following page. Your activity can be anything from walking, workouts, or a sport. Rate your performance from 1-10 for each corresponding week.

Copy This Page - On a Copy Machine

Activity 1._____Date_____

Activity 2._____Date_____

Activity 3._____Date_____

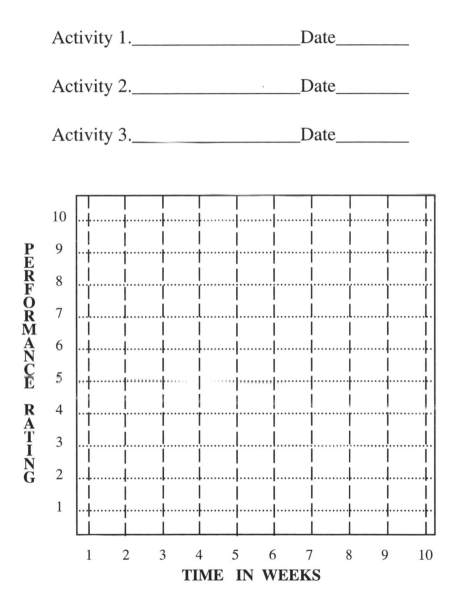

This Activity Chart Name_____

Quite often, when people enter into a self-improvement program they miss one of the key elements for success in the program, which is the measuring stick. Or in some cases, they use the wrong measuring stick. The most common example of this is people who go on diets to lose weight and use a scale as their measuring stick. Uninformed, they consider that their problem is weight. Of course, in many cases it is, but more to the point, their real problem is their fat-to-body mass ratio. So what they should be measuring is their fat count and not their weight. The same concept can be applied to postural therapy via the Symmetry Program.

Postural problems can be quite subtle and difficult to detect. So, if you're going strictly for improvements in posture and alignment, you might find your gains difficult to measure. This is why it is very helpful to utilize one of your favorite physical activities as the measuring stick for improvement. Even if the activity is as simple as walking, you may notice that on some days walking is easier or more satisfying than others. More strenuous or complicated activities, such as skiing, golf, tennis, biking, running or other sports, are easier to measure based on performance and potentially, competition. If you are no longer involved in an activity or sport that you used to enjoy, it may well be that a postural problem has led to your inactivity. That is the subtlety of postural problems -- you may not be aware that you have them. As a matter of fact, most people are unaware that they have postural problems and further, they're unaware of the long-term ill effects.

For now, to make the concept of a performance evaluation easier to envision, let's use a weekend golfer for our model. Postural therapy and golf go hand in hand and many of the world's greatest golfers practice the principles and exercises to maintain postural therapy. Obviously, if your back, shoulders and hips are misaligned, the activity of swinging a golf club will be inconsistent at best. This is the beauty of using golf as an example for the benefits of postural therapy and a performance evaluation. Almost every aspect of the game of golf can be improved with correct postural alignment: strength, striking distance, accuracy, touch and endurance are all affected and potentially corrected with proper postural alignment.

Take It One Step at a Time

When you begin to prepare your performance evaluation, take one aspect at a time or you may become overwhelmed by the process. Perhaps the best place to start is with the golf swing. When a golfer's swing is improved, so is most of his or her game, so this is an important part of the evaluation. If a golfer were to look at a chart starting from when he or she began the game to where he or she is now, there should be a steady line of improvement for a period of time. At some point things might begin to level off or get worse.

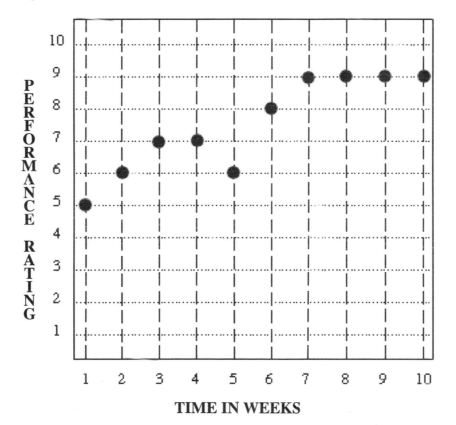

TIME IN WEEKS

Here the performance started at an average level, improved, dipped and finally evened out with a "9" rating. This person felt that his performance had room for improvement, hence the "9" rating.

In Summary

You are motivated to make a change in your life and are looking for relief and/or self- improvement. If that were not the case, you would never have made it to the summary, right? An honest evaluation is the key to getting started on an improvement in motion dynamics and pain relief. If the problem is pain, take a look at your routines that lead to the pain and the methods you use to relieve the pain. If the pain keeps coming back, then you have perpetuating factors which, until challenged, will continue to cause habitual pain. For those who are involved in a sport and wonder why they don't seem to be making the type of improvements desired, again evaluation is the key. Look at the chart and distinguish the causes and effects of improvement vs. stagnation. You can use charts as tools to help gauge your successes in sports or to chart the onset, causes and perpetuating factors of pain.

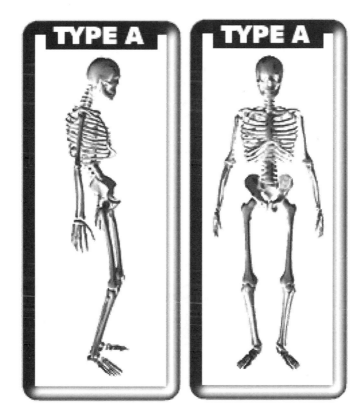

A Perfect World Vs. Reality

The fact that life is an ongoing process gives pause on occasion for those considering the need for self-improvement programs. All self-improvement programs are based upon changes and techniques, so if you're going to change something, it helps if you know why the change is necessary in the first place. Should you go along with the program verbatim, or take the program on your own terms? Without a doubt, self-improvement programs require a willingness to make the changes necessary for success. In many cases, people take change or directions on blind faith for time's sake or out of desperation. Since this program is a lifestyle concept, time is on your side and there is no reason to rush or desperately reach ahead for results, because there is no way to access how fast you will achieve your desired results. Some people will experience positive results almost immediately, while others have to work at it on a daily basis for the rest of their lives.

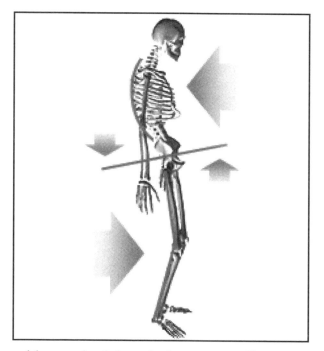

Sitting with your back hunched can cause tilted hips and a "C" curve in the back. This position leads to dysfunctional and fluctuating movement.

As we mentioned in the last chapter, most of the problems that people experience with performance and perpetual pain are based around habits that force the body into compromising situations. As children experience movement and function as part of a daily routine, they take situations head-on without much regard for outcome. They have not been programmed to understand what actions cause pain and what situations could create problems for them in the future. On the other hand, adults flinch, pull back, and stop short throughout their day, causing various muscle and bone problems. Simply put, adults are tentative in their movements and execute caution based on perceptions and programming accumulated during their lives. Many adults believe that if they move too fast they might get hurt, or if they move too slowly, they might not get out of the way fast enough. Tenuous movement, unnecessary caution and muscular isolation are almost the exact opposite of how children move throughout their day. As an example, if you were to observe the posture, positioning and movement of ten preschool children playing kick ball compared to ten thirty-year-olds play-

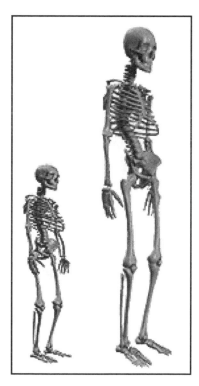

ing, you would see an example of a perfect world versus reality.

From a physical standpoint, children live in a near-perfect world. Their posture is good. They have no accumulated physical trauma or injury which may lead to perpetuating pain factors. Children are also not overly cautious.

As people mature they often develop a slanted pelvis and a rounded back from sitting or poor postural habits. Children generally start life in nearly perfect alignment.

Teaching a child to ski is much easier than teaching an adult who is filled with fear and trepidation. So we use the model of a child as the basis for a perfect world and compare that to the reality that adults choose to live in. The keyword is choose — meaning adults choose to live in whatever world they decide. By comparison, children don't choose their environment — they are thrown into activities, and yet their actions, movements and dynamics are generally healthy and vigorous. Without training, the body does what's right for it, but with experience and social input, natural choices are overridden by conscious decisions. Such decisions are the realities by which adults live and move. In a perfect world, you do what's fun and you do what you like, but in the real world choices are no longer purely individual.

Let's look at some examples of how children live in a world that perpetuates positive structural, physical development and enables postural stability. Based on natural fact, children are in constant growth and change patterns and they observe that things don't come as easily for them as they do for the adults that they watch. They see adults playing basketball outside in the street and they know they lack the strength to shoot a basket. This knowledge sets them free because they know that no matter how hard they try, they can't make a basket until they are a little bigger. They're not embarrassed, they don't have to worry about form following function and they know they look silly and get a laugh when they drop the ball. But reality sets in for the adults when the few who are in shape decide to go for a quick pick-up basketball game. If they decide not to play, they will be looked down upon by some, and if they want to play but feel that they can't, they may be subconsciously admitting that they are getting too old. Reality in today's world says that you can fight getting old and delay the aging process. But you've got to have the necessary tools.

Building and Tools

If you were to give a child a box full of parts that needed to be assembled to make a table, you would see just how physical the process can be. Several things would be observed, not to mention the possible comedy that would ensue right from the start. Almost every action the child took to complete the task would be unnecessary from the viewpoint of an experienced adult. Since the child would have no experience with tools, he wouldn't automatically look for tools, especially power tools to expedite the process. Instead he would mill about and try virtually every conceivable combination and idea imaginable for him. The process would be very physically demanding because all the tools he would have to work with would be the original equipment from birth. Hands, arms, legs, back — would all be working nonstop in a flurry of activity; nothing tentative, caution cast aside, damn the torpedoes — here I come. As a result, the child would experience a good workout, do some stretching and develop some new hand-eye coordination.

One of the most interesting features noted while watching a child in action is how he or she holds themselves throughout an activity. They are typically upright and move using 90-degree angle body positions. They don't take shortcuts regarding motion, and don't reach for objects, but rather get up and move toward the object. In short, children are not afraid or intimidated in any way concerning their movements and dynamics in action. They are motion machines, and as a result, almost everything about their physical dynamics works better and more efficiently to serve their needs as they see them. Watching children play kick ball and observing them in line waiting for their turn to kick, one sees that they're moving with erect posture and straight backs. When it is their turn to kick the ball, they run to the ball with poor timing, but still follow through without conscious regard of outcome. Conversely, when adults stand in line waiting for their turn to kick the ball, they are in a slouched position, head down, holding still with tilted hips, knees, and shoulders. When it is their turn to kick the ball they often approach the ball tentatively and do not follow through with their kick. They run cautiously and do not extend their arms or legs like the children. Most adults seem to have lost at least fifty percent of the range of motion that the children demonstrate.

Most adults look for the most efficient way to complete a task. If you were to give a table kit that required assembly to an adult, the first thing they would do is look for a proper workspace. If available, they would look for an area with a workbench to begin the assembly process. Prior to assembling the table, they would gather any and all tools available to make a job go faster and easier. There would be as little movement as possible and virtually no new development with hand-eye coordination. The adult would make the process as easy as possible, requiring as little movement as necessary, which is the exact opposite of the child. Certainly the adult would do a better job of assembling the table, but the child would do a better job of developing his or her body and hand-eye coordination. So at the end of the day, who really did a better job, the child or the adult?

A child's unnecessary motion has the cumulative effect of strengthening the body and motion dynamics at large. An adult's conservation of movement has the cumulative effect of softening muscles and decreasing the range of motion. Because of the differences in a sedentary life compared to the perpetual motion of a child, adults eventually must return to physical activities or greatly suffer the consequences. The consequences become the most apparent when an adult is put in a situation which requires a new range of motion. Since a child's world is all motion, there isn't much new that they could experience in the world of motion dynamics that they don't experience on a daily basis in play. Children roll around on the floor, they are constantly picking themselves up from a fall, and all their parts are moving in a full range of motion every day. The concept of conserving energy is simply not part of their routine. Children go until they drop. After a nap with recharged batteries, they're up and going.

Learn to Imitate Children

If children live in a perfect world regarding the dynamics of motion, ever developing hand-eye coordination, miraculous healing rates, no pulled muscles and no headaches, shouldn't we take notice of their lifestyle? Even if you ask a child to watch a television program or work at a computer station, you'll notice that they get up, move around, stretch out and change positions constantly. They do not conserve energy, and as a result they have more energy than their adult counterparts. The intriguing concept is that the more energy you burn, the more energy you have available. This is what children do — this is their lifestyle, and in retrospect their world is truly a wonder. The question is, what can adults do to bring themselves back to the health, vigor and energy enjoyed by children?

If motion is the key to health, vitality and energy, then why do adults constantly look for a means to conserve motion? There are probably many ways to answer that question, but one of the most obvious answers points to social and cultural status. This is where the trouble for adults begins, in that society often looks down on those whose jobs are more physically demanding. Notwithstanding the recent cultural boom of professional athletics, people who work with their hands have been titled blue-collar workers and experience lower scales of pay. Here again we battle with the perfect world vs. reality, where, in a perfect or child-like world, our social and economic status would not decline as a result of physical tenacity at work. Those less physically challenged by work are considered to be in managerial positions or experiencing more luxury. As luxury is considered desirable and certainly marketed as such, its desired attributes become the reality that ignites the debilitating lack of motion that goes with the lifestyle.

What is considered more luxurious, a television with a remote control or a television without a remote control? Even a child can answer that question: because with a remote you don't have to move to change channels on the television. Which is considered superior in this society, a hand saw or power saw? When was the last time you saw somebody drill a hole with a mechanical hand drill? I don't think my children have ever seen a mechanical hand drill. So our desire to obtain a higher social status often creates a reality that includes a receding and sometimes paralyzing range of motion. But an interesting thing has happened regarding the world of luxury: youth and a youthful range of motion and dynamics are now considered attributes of the socially elite.

When I grew up in the '60's and '70's, the adults would come home from a hard day's work, rest, eat dinner and rest some more. During the weekends — weather permitting — I would see parents working in their yards and even on their cars. Gardeners and mechanics were often the luxuries that the American middle-class could not even consider. Also, mothers were not working in the workplace as they are today. After a hard day of working in the yard, on the car or whatever, the adults I knew would relax with friends and neighbors mostly sitting, eating and relaxing. Today's modern luxuries and salaries have created a new service industry for the modern middle class. Those living within the middle class, and certainly those with means beyond the middle class, enjoy services including painters, gardeners, mechanics, maid services, daycare assistance and even home-delivered, cooked meals. So, since many people are able to utilize such services, what do they do with all of their spare time? The answer: play like children. Today's adults want to play like children and this is a relatively new social development.

Toys For Adult Tots

Children are not the only ones with toys these days. Many adults have more toys than their children because manufacturers are making them available and marketing them aggressively. Also, there are more activity clubs and adult sports leagues than ever before. Adults are learning to play hockey by the millions, and hockey is a very physically demanding sport. Adults are learning to ski and roller blade, which both require an advanced level of coordination, strength, and flexibility to remain injury-free. There is now gymnastics for adults, and even bungle jumping for seniors, so now it seems that everyone wants to act young again.

So what happens when a relatively inactive, hard-working adult decides to revisit the days of his hyperactive childhood? Simple: pain and injury are the result when heretofore inactive adults jump into childhood activities. The truth is that no one wants to grow old with grace in a stationary dynamic. Now with the help of advertising agencies, adults are fighting age tooth and nail with every fiber of their being. If you are not among the active, you are considered either unhealthy or not financially stable enough to participate in the activities. So now the choices are far different than they were just one generation ago — get on the activity bus or grow old alone.

Issues Leading to Self-Diagnosis

In the first few chapters of this book, the initial concepts were to help you understand how habits, circumstances and stagnation lead to pain and less-than-ideal dynamics of motion. This next section is the starting block that will hopefully lead you down the right path. The good news about the diagnosis procedure is that the issue can be black and white. First, you'll note whether or not your posture is ideal or if it is great, but if it's not, what category do you fit into? There are no great mysteries here, so be confident that the information about your self-diagnosis will be easy to digest and understand.

If pain, muscular dysfunction, and less-than-ideal dynamics in motion are signals that you need help, then a self-diagnosis would be the best place to start. In the science of postural therapy, there are three main categories of physical alignment conditions. In most cases, your body type and postural positioning will fit very closely to one of the three basic conditions. If your body type and alignment are nearly ideal based on the model of the ideal postural alignment body, then we will have to look a little closer at specific areas that might be slightly in opposition. If you were to consider a goal at this point, it would be to have a body with all the right angles and horizontal lines in correct alignment. We could call a person with perfect alignment a "P. A.," and to become more familiar with how rare a P. A. is, you will be excited when you see one. Of course, if you want to see them by the dozens, go to a playground and watch a bunch of four-year-olds running and playing.

Just like any other tool, the human body has a function, and naturally it performs better when its parts are aligned and prepared to work as designed. You can imagine that when any tool, such as a hammer, has a handle that is bent or a chipped and broken head, it won't drive nails very well. In fact, a hammer in that condition would probably become even more damaged when you tried to use it. That is exactly what happens to the human body when its parts are out of alignment and it is unprepared to do the work that it is asked to do.

If you can look at the average person and try to guess what will they do and what won't they do with their body, then you can develop a basis for dynamic measurement. You could look at two older women, perhaps in their late 70's, and one of them might be stooped and bent, while the other is upright and spry. Maybe they're both the at grocery store and you notice that one of them asks for assistance quite often, while the other can reach both up and down to get anything she wants off the shelf. Further, you might wonder how the lady with less dynamic motion handles stairs, getting in and out of cars and even how she opens heavy doors. The key thing to note is what type of postural alignment differences you can observe between the two ladies. Now, because you don't know them, you can make an honest evaluation of their posture, at least from your perspective. The trick is, can you do the same thing with yourself when you stand in front of the mirror?

Now let's get back to the subject of you and what you can do with your body. As we've mentioned earlier, compared to children, most adults seem relatively motionless. Of course, we all know that our hearts beat, our lungs expand and contract; our circulatory system runs like a highway, so even when we're sitting still our bodies are in constant motion. Unfortunately, involuntary movement doesn't count when it comes to postural alignment and dynamics of motion. Your musculoskeletal structure needs a conscious effort from you to work properly. Another bit of complicating news is that your involuntary system needs assistance from your voluntary muscles in order to move blood, transfer oxygen throughout your body and replenish the nervous system. So whether you want to or not, you have to move and stay in motion or suffer the consequences.

Gravity and Movement

The purpose of this book is to help people get out of pain and improve their overall health through dynamics of motion. This is done by teaching the body how to cope with today's modern lifestyles. If you want success you not only have to cope with an extremely fast-paced, high stress environment, but you also have to master motion. Success cannot be achieved unless you learn to master your dynamics and mastery demands high productivity and high-performance with the limited resources of time that are available. Conceptually you have to do much more with much less time than previously allowed while meeting our day-to-day deadlines.

We also hope that this book helps to dispel myths and help people understand the source of their pain. Many go to the gym three times a week and watch what they eat, but as a society they need to understand that it is not activity that counts, but correct activity. Going to the gym utilizes the gross muscle groups, not the deep postural muscles that maintain correct skeletal function. Our bodies need the correct stimulus to prevent body pain. Doing exercises and lifting weights in the wrong positions can often stimulate compensating muscles which should not be used in the first place. Compensating muscles do the work for muscles that have become atrophyed due to an injury or poor postural alignment.

Another myth is that age can be the cause of body pain, but pain does not know age. It is time that causes the body to break down so that, as time progresses we learn to get away with fewer useless movements. It is not that we are any healthier as children, merely that time had not yet taken its total on the body. Combining the factor of time with insufficient or incorrect stimulus is one of the major causes of body pain.

Pain is extremely objective and our bodies know that they have pain. What they do not understand is why pain seeks a specific area of the body. The concept of symmetry is to focus on the cause of pain not the symptom. This can be done in three steps: evaluation, pain alleviation and education.

Without question, we have become the product of modernization. We live in and age when technology forces us to sit for long periods of time often in front of computers. There are great financial rewards for tenacity and poignant work ethic, but the setbacks are obvious and are well-documented for the last two decades. But the workplace is just where the sitting starts, and consider how we get to work, via seated transportation and what happens after work sitting at dinner or in from the TV.

Sitting weakens the muscles designed to keep our body in the correct position around gravity. If the muscles are no longer able to hold the correct body position pain will ensue. There should be no mystery about this concept if you consider what group of people are most likely to experience chronic pain. When do people begin to get headaches? Interestingly, children don't get a lot of headaches, and the reason for this is that their bodies are being used for the purpose they are intended — which is movement. When movement is consistent and repetitive the body will rejuvenate itself and the processes of healing are not necessary. But when a person is stagnant the muscles learn to stay short and the tendons learn to maintain a short range of motion. And then as new movement or strenuous movement is required an injury will quickly occur.

Gravity is the main culprit in causing body pain because our bodies are exposed to tremendous pressures bearing down. We are born with a concept of gravity and don't question it, but very few people realize the extent of the force of gravity. The reason this is significant is because our bodies are designed to maintain themselves in gravity in a very specific way. Our joints are meant to lineup with the same line as gravity. Gravity moves in a straight line which can be evidenced by watching an object fall straight to the ground.

Our modern lifestyle forces our bodies out of alignment as we hunch and stoop in seated positions throughout our busy day. Our deep postural muscles are the foundation for proper alignment and the dysfunction of these muscles knocks our skeleton out of its proper position. Incorrect body alignment causes compensation, which is when different muscles are used to fill the function of weakened muscles. It is this compensation that can be targeted as a main cause for body pain. The constant force of gravity allows us no forgiveness of dysfunction and therefore gravity becomes our enemy. So the main physical property which is responsible for our strength can also be a liability if ignored for long periods of time.

Let's Have a Look at Back Pain

Do you have body pain? If you answered yes to this question, you're not alone. Today, 35 million Americans suffer from some type of back or joint pain. The inevitable question that must be asked is why? In this age of modern specialization's why do we endure chronic pain without the benefit of long-term relief? To answer these questions one must understand the human body as it relates to its environment.

Pain is a creation of modern society and our contemporary lifestyle. Our ancestors spent their days in constant activity. They ran, jumped, and hunted. This constant demand forced postural and structural muscles to develop as they were intended. Their natural lifestyle maintained the postural integrity of their bodies.

Today, on the other hand, we inhibit our bodies' natural motion through our dependence on modern transportation, technology and automation. Ninety percent of our time is spent sitting, moving, or operating in ways our bodies were not intended. We wake-up, drive to work, and sit in front of a computer for hours, then come home and sit in front of the television. Even when making deliberate attempts to exercise, we tend towards programs that work against our bodies natural motion, placing emphasis on burning calories and building muscle, not on facilitating full range of motion and unrestricted movement. Muscles designed for vital functions, such as bending, twisting, and lifting shut down. Other muscles not intended for these functions must fill in for them, thus compensation occurs. It is this compensation — the result of not using our bodies as they were intended, which causes pain. What we labeled "inevitable aging," genetics, or "just the way we are" is simply the consequence of a failure to prevent system breakdown.

To understand more about system breakdown, however, we must first understand postural integrity as it relates to our bodies design. Right angles form at the shoulder, hip, knee and ankle joints and support us structurally. Our spinal column is composed of individual vertebrae, each capable of four degrees of movement, front and back. This movement facilitates equal weight distribution from head to toe, forming the basis of parallel and vertical lines. These right angles enable us to have bilateral function. Symmetry — we have two hands, two arms, two feet, two legs. Our left and right sides are designed to do the same things. We are intended to function as a unit, a whole. We are in essence the sum of our parts. There's great strength in this bilateral function, but also weakness: if just one part of the whole decides to function incorrectly, the integrity of the whole is jeopardized, and we have pain.

So where does the pain come from? As your heel strikes, a functional muscle evenly distributes the shock to the joints and sockets. Imagine that there is a body dysfunction causing compensation — the wrong muscle moving the wrong bone into the wrong position. As the heel strikes, the shock is not evenly distributed to the joints, but is focused on specific points, abrading cartilage, tendon, ligament or bone. With this constant repetition occurring in the absence of a symmetrical, efficient whole, individual parts deteriorate and then breakdown. This is when your body screams. "This is not working! This is not right!" The way we hcar is through pain. Pain, therefore is the symptom and not the problem.

There is a way to address the real problem. If treating the symptom is like putting sand bags around a broken dam, then how can you prevent the dam from continually breaking? Very simply — you rebuild the dam. Through a series of specific postural exercises, the body can be retrained to function according to its original design. First you must educate muscle to hold bone correctly. This circumvents the need for continual treatment and once your body is structurally strong, you are able to maintain this strength through the daily reinforcement of proper exercise. Second, use your bodies own natural antagonism to provide resistance. Avoid reliance on equipment and let gravity be your friend and not your enemy. Third, address your body as a unit. You must be able to a identify the source of your body pain. Once identified, you can target and reduce your pain's source through a systematic process of individualized postural exercises. If you never find the source, you'll never truly be satisfied. You can return to a healthy, functional lifestyle. With an emphasis on education and evaluation, you can be provided with tools necessary to be self-sufficient in this age of "quick fixes." Part of this process is learning the know-how and understanding that it is never too late to turn back the clock.

Learning to Be Young Again

Have you ever looked into a mirror and really focused on your body? Besides the occasional bad hair day, have you ever noticed anything unusual about the way your body looks posturally? Over 35 million people suffer from back or joint pain today in America, and the quick fix is no longer a viable option to solving the problem. Taking drugs or adjusting the symptom is like knocking the fire alarm off the ceiling in the middle of the night because it annoys you then two hours later you wake-up to a burning house.

So what does posture have to do with curing your pain? Let's go back to the mirror again. Your body was designed like the children you see playing outside — symmetrical. Compare yourself to a child and notice the differences. There is a basic design we were all intended to have and maintain. The problem is not that we get older, it is that we are no longer as active as the children we see playing everyday and can no longer maintain our original design. When our designed system breaks down, the body lets us know. By helping our body return back to its intended design, a new healthy way of life can be achieved. We sit 70 percent of the day, so maintaining postural strength and positioning is the key to living without pain. The answers all exist as you stand in front of the mirror, so take a good look and consider how your posture compares to a four-year old child.

The Main Objective

You can maintain and enhance optimal health and function through neuro-muscular reeducation by teaching muscles to hold bones in their correct positions. Muscles have a functional memory and once the muscles are trained to hold bone positions correctly, optimal postural health can become a reality.

The process of postural therapy is individualistic such that each person has a varying degrees of postural problems. For this reason it is difficult to gauge how long the process of postural therapy will take to fix a pain or condition. Some people experience nearly complete results in just one session by positioning and exercising their body in a way that their posture reacts too quickly. Yet in other cases, a sequence of exercises must be completed for the final desired results. Think of it like taking the skin off all of an onion, there could be several layers of muscle that need to be addressed in a particular sequential manner. The sequences, exercises and finally the amount of time it will take to experience the desired results are based upon an honest evaluation. You must gauge how you compare to nature's original design. The further out of alignment you are, the longer it will take you to correct the postural problem. The key points are that postural conditions are correctable, and that postural therapy corrects conditions that cause less than desirable performance and symptoms of pain.

If you were to schedule a postural therapy treatment session, the session could last about eight weeks. Initially the session would start with a diagnosis and then work into an exercise sequence with follow-up diagnoses. Other aspects of the session would include de-programming, which refers to the habits, movements and aspects of your lifestyle which contribute to postural problems. In some cases it may be understood that certain aspects of movement should cease in order to benefit from treatment. Naturally age, height, weight, condition, and general physical attributes will play into the process. The main focus and goal in any postural therapy program is the understanding that regardless of other physical conditions each individual has a best case postural scenario. It is this best case that you should attempt to achieve.

Your body needs to learn how to readjust to living conditions and new stimuli generated from the exercise programs. You also need to recondition yourself mentally to maintain proper postural integrity throughout your day. Simply becoming aware of postural problems often helps to consciously change body positions and stimulate proper movement. Soon muscles that were not used to maintaining proper posture will commence action and muscles that

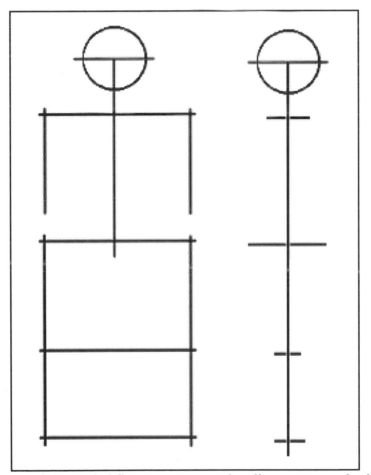

These right angled figures represent the alignment your body was meant to maintain. This is not an exaggeration.

were compensating for improper posture will go back to doing the work for which they were intended by nature.

Gauge Yourself at Home

One of the most important aspects of this program is the Self-Diagnosis. You'll need to perform and honest evaluation on yourself to help gauge your postural status. Your body was designed to operate with joints at 90 degree angles. Your shoulders should be 90 degrees to your chest bone and your spine should be 90 degrees to your hips. Your legs should attach to your hips at 90 degree

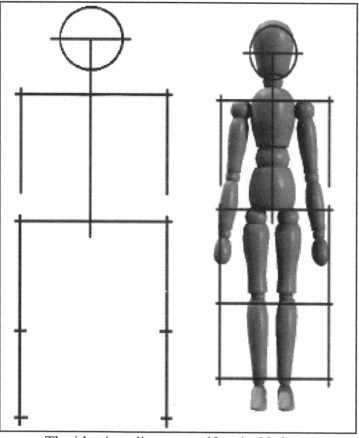

The idea is to line yourself up in 90 degree
angles such as shown here...

angles and so on. 90 degrees is the basic concept on which postural therapy is built. Interestingly, your body is also built on 90 degree angles. Motion is performed optimally when a human body is straight and contoured with 90 degree angles.

Tie a string to a ceiling or top of a doorway with a weight of some kind hanging from the bottom of it. This is called a plum line, and represents a straight line of gravity. One of the easiest ways to make a plumb line is to take a piece of string and tie a one inch metal washer to the bottom of it. Tack the top of the string to the top of a door-way, and now you are in business. Postural therapists use a plumb line to determine how a patient measures up with a straight line. It is best if you can find a way to hang a plumb line in front of a mirror so you can see yourself and the plumb line in the mirror at the same time. The very best case scenario is to have another person take a picture of you from both sides front and back while comparing your posture alignment to a plumb line.

You could also use a video camera and rotate yourself in align-

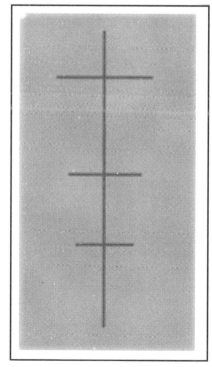

If you have a full length mirror, then your are in business.

Draw this pattern, but try to keep the lines straight. You could always use a wall with a washable marker of some type... Don't permenently mark your walls!

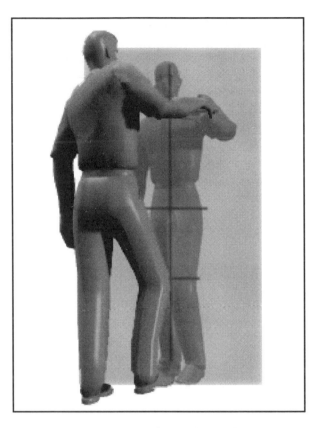

**A full length mirror is perfect so
you can see yourself and the lines.**

ment with a plum line showing front, back and side views. If you
feel so inclined, another very good method is to use a full-length
mirror and a "white board" erasable marker to create a "posture
map." The trick is to make certain that your angles are true and
correct. If you have a t-square use it to make perfect 90 degree
angles. Draw a big "T" on the mirror. Line yourself up so the top
of the T matches up with your shoulders. Once you have your self
aligned in the mirror, mark the spot where you were standing so
you can go back to that spot again. The next idea is to draw three
more lines which cross the long plum line. You'll want to draw a
line where your hips would match on the mirror from your marked

standing position, and another line for your knees and your ankles.

Your drawing of the T on the mirror should now have a total of floor 90 degree lines intersect it. From the top to bottom the lines should match with your shoulder line, hip line, knee line and ankles. You should stand with your shoes off and preferably in as little clothing as possible so none of your postural positions will be covered. Typically a bathing suit works fine, but if you can go with no clothes on at all, even better. Of course the naked diagnosis, is for your own personal education. No pictures or videos are necessary for this type of personal diagnosis.

If you have someone that can help you chart your postural positions, then there are a few extra things you can do to get a more realistic and professional personal evaluation. First align yourself

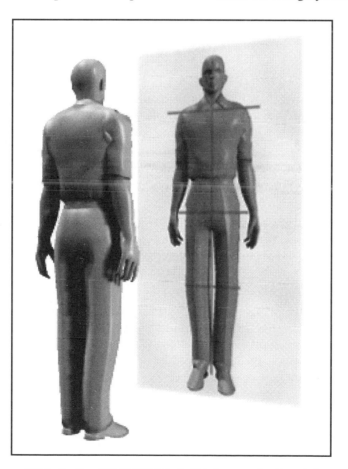

This is the RIGHT idea, Right angle that is!

with the plumb line running between your eyes, through the middle of your chest, and straight between your knees and ankles. In other words, line yourself up as best as possible with a plumb line. Now closed your eyes, raise your arms up over your head slowly and then lower them down to your sides slowly. Take two slow motion marching steps in place be careful to maintain your foot position and alignment with the plumb line. Remember to keep your eyes closed during this process. The object here is to find the most honest diagnostic position alignment possible, that will not be affected or subconsciously corrected by you viewing yourself in comparison to the plumb line. Technically you could perform the same type of diagnosis by yourself and then open your eyes without moving to compare yourself to lines it drawn on the mirror.

The purpose of this is self diagnostic postural review is to create a comparison chart. Obviously a person needs to know where they are starting from regarding their postural alignment. After doing a few exercises some people experience an improved postural alignment immediately. After training the muscles and your mind to maintain correct postural positions, you'll find your overall postural gauge to be vastly improved. In fact simply looking at the mirror and honestly evaluating your posture will greatly serve to motivate you to a better postural positioning. This is not a onetime fix all, but rather a lifetime concept. Once you have mastered the perception of correct posture alignment, you will subconsciously strive to maintain correct posture.

The trick to getting an honest postural alignment evaluation is to get your hips into action before settling into a still position. The alignment of the hips is what dictates the position of the feet and often the shoulders and back. If the hips are tilted front to back or back to front, the back will be swayed or slumped to compensate. If the hips are tilted to one side or another, then the knees will compensate. So when you are doing your evaluation, marching in slow motion in place with your eyes closed will help to give you and honest position without the bias of eye site.

COPY THIS PAGE

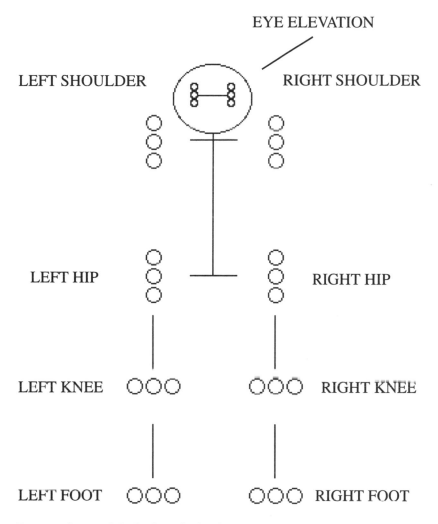

Instructions: Mark the circle that you most closely line up with, and remember, be honest with your posture.
For example is one shoulder higher or lower than center? Is one side of your hips higher or lower? Do your feet and knees point straight ahead or aim in or out a little?

Theoretically you can use any right angle to line up against or compare to. There are several things inside a house or apartment that are right angle such as door jams, the corner of a wall running from floor to ceiling or anything that has an edge perpendicular to a floor or ceiling. The reason hanging a plum line works so well is because that it gets you into the spirit of perfect alignment by actually lining something up yourself. When you go through the physical steps of lining up and hanging a plum line, you gather a sense of what perfect alignment is as well as what it looks and feels like. You might think of it this way; hanging a plum line gets you in the mood for correct postural alignment. You get a string, tie a weight to the bottom of it and hang it from the ceiling or doorway. It swings for a second or two, and when it stops, it is perfectly aligned. Your eye will subconsciously compare it to other things that may not be lined up as well. Since you'll be hanging the plumb line in consideration of a comparison of your own posture alignment, you'll instantly sense areas in your own body that could be out of alignment. So this is why we recommend using your own plumb line instead of something else that might be a right angle in your home.

Hidden Postural Messages

In some cases you might not have a mirror or someone to help you with a plumb line. You'll have to become your own detective to attempt to diagnose potential postural problems. For example if your legs hurt, note whether or not your knees are pointing forward. You might find that one knee is higher than another or that one knee is pointing a little bit to the left or right. Perhaps your legs are slightly bowed or maybe one ankle is positioned differently than the other. These are hidden postural messages and ways that your bones and muscles compensate for pains and misalignment. Just like a car, if one tire is out of alignment, the other tires will compensate by wearing unevenly. As a result, the tires will eventually wear faster and become damaged more easily, and your body is no different.

It often helps to think of your body as a machine that was designed for movement. Some machines are made to operate in stationary positions. Typically televisions, stereos and computers are made to operate from stationery positions. Naturally there are some moving parts, but the unit itself is made to operate from a standard still position. But audio cassette players and video players have several moving parts which if not exercised regularly will literally degrade. If you let a video player or tape player set for too long, it's plastic and rubber belt parts will rot and break. Quite often people are amazed when such an electronic component doesn't work even though they haven't used it for a long period of time. They wonder how it could be broken after so little use. The answer is "dry rot." Rubber and plastic parts need to be moved. Quite often they are lubricated for life at the factory, and as they are used the lubricants spread evenly over the entire part. Steady movement keeps a part lubricated and ready for action. The human body is made of parts that need to be moved for optimal usage.

When a Body Is Stagnant It Degrades

The point of stagnation cannot be driven home hard enough. Think of it this way: "Hold Still and Break." When you fall down, your body is made to get right back up. But if you've been holding still and stagnant in your lifestyle for a long period of time, getting right back up might be a problem. That's why I say "if you hold still long enough, you'll break."

Try to imagine what would happen in a boxing match if one of the boxers was to stand or sit in the same position relatively still for an hour before the match. Picture a boxing ring. In one corner is a boxer who is running in place working his neck, arms and shoulders. In the other corner is a boxer sitting in a lounge chair with his feet up watching TV. The bell sounds. One boxer is ready for anything. The other boxer snaps to his feet and is instantly dizzy. The ready boxer throws one little punch and the stagnant boxer falls back in his lounge chair, dazed and confused. The act of simply getting up is difficult if not impossible. Getting out of the way of a punch was completely out of question.

Be Ready for Anything

Physical injuries occur because people are not ready to adjust to the actions or contortions placed on their bodies in a certain instant. If your body is ready for anything, then it can adjust to anything. I heard about a story of one lady who was getting her hair done. She was setting in a chair with the dryer running for about forty-five minutes. She stood up when the drying was finished stepped down from the chair and broke both of her legs. I have remembered this story ever since, and have always thought about how important it is to make sure that my body is ready to move when I am.

Weekend Warriors are the athletes who sit around all week and then run out to play tennis, football or softball. Their flexibility is

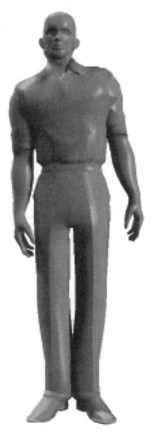

How could you ever expect to move consistently when your shoulders rotate incorrectly? Try to swing a golf club, tennis racket, baseball bat, or even swim straight when your body is pointing in the wrong direction. Correct this problem and watch some incredible new consistency come into your dynamics of motion.

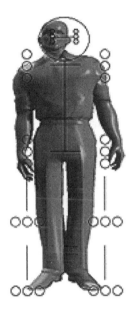

anything but optimal and their strength is certainly in question for the tasks they are requesting of their body. They run to first base and sprain their knee or ankle. In some cases the injury can be far more serious and discs in the back can be broken or shocked out of alignment. You have to move. If you don't you will get sick or injured. That's all there is to it. I had a backup CD player that I almost never used. It had a few different rubber belts that connected to sprockets which would in turn spin the CD at the correct speed. It had been sitting in a closet when after about a year I pulled it out for party. I turned the CD player on, placed a CD on the tray, and pressed the play button. The unit simply wouldn't work. The second I hit the play button, the play belt jammed and then damaged the laser reader. The two hundred dollar machine was broken just because I had not used it. There are two morals to the story:
1. Don't buy a CD player that you're not going to use.
2. Don't attempt a physical task unless you're realistically ready.

Think of Postural Alignment As Insurance

Everyone has heard that you shouldn't try something that you are not ready for, but you do it anyway. If you have correct postural alignment, then your body is almost ready for anything. Maybe you're not as flexible as you should be and maybe you're not as strong as you should be,

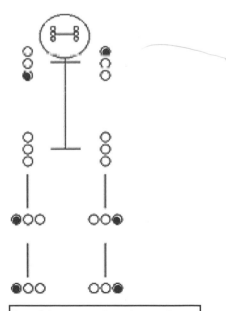

In this sample chart from above one shoulder is up; the other is down. Also the knees and feet both point outward.

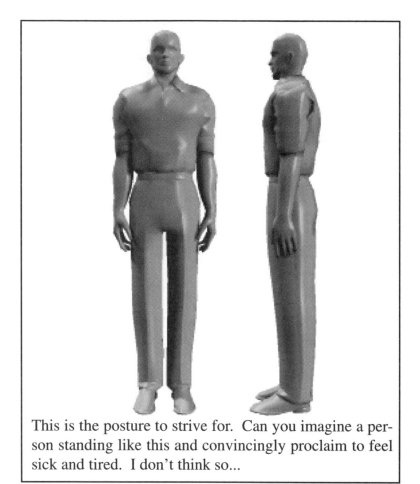

This is the posture to strive for. Can you imagine a person standing like this and convincingly proclaim to feel sick and tired. I don't think so...

but at least your body will be in the right position when you swing into action. Having correct postural alignment takes some work and a little discipline, but once you get there, maintaining it can become nearly automatic.

When your body is positioned erect and straight you are more apt and prepared to fight off difficulties and daily stress. When you are slumped over, your body and emotional feelings are prone to take in the physical burdens of daily turmoil and stress. It's hard to stand straight and erect with shoulders back and chest out and say, "I feel rotten." Conversely, it is also hard to say, "I feel great" when your shoulders are slumped over and your chest is sunken and withdrawn.

The Integration of Posture and Emotion

There seems to be a significant relationship between the way the human body holds itself posturally and emotions. The relationship can work one of two ways in that either emotions manifest themselves in posture or posture manifests emotions.

Regardless of the relationship regarding the integration of posture and emotion, there is little doubt that positive posture serves to fight off stress and creates more health serving emotions. This particular subject could be an entire book unto itself but that is not our purpose here. Our purpose is to quickly glance over certain aspects of human life which can be improved with enhanced posture.

Again it's important to note for our purposes here, that posture does not simply refer to how straight your back and shoulders are. When we talk about posture, we're considering the entire aspect and physiology regarding postural therapy as a whole. We consider the hips, back, shoulders, neck, legs, feet and even arms and hands. Furthermore, we consider the aspect of compensation as the key and source of the majority of pains often manifested as postural ailments.

In consideration of the concept that posture is fully integrated and effects the bodies systems on the whole, all the following must be considered as potential targets for sickness or poor health:

Emotional
Neurological
Circulatory
Respiratory
Digestive

As is mentioned above, emotional considerations can be played out from one of two directions, emotions creating postural ailments or postural ailments creating unhealthful emotions.

Neurological disorders are obviously related in some manner to postural malody's. People with poor posture or other postural disorders suffer pain, and pain is reported via neurological systems to the brain.

The circulatory system can be regarded as integrated with postural considerations much the same as the neurological system. Sitting incorrectly also decreases optimal circulation as does any less than optimal postural positioning. Basic common sense would suggest that and optimal postural position would enhance blood flow and circulation.

The respiratory system and lung capacity in general is greatly affected by the position and posture of the shoulders, back and hips if the hips tilt incorrectly the back can be thrown out of alignment pushing shoulders down in a slumped position. This slumped position decreases the amount of chest expansion and therefore the amount of oxygen that can be drawn into the lungs from breathing. Smaller breaths means smaller air intake and less oxygen which leads to less energy and potentially depressed emotional feelings.

The digestive system is affected in much the same way as the respiratory system with regard to poor postural positioning. Slumped positioning cramps intestines, the stomach, and the colon. Once again common sense should be followed regarding posture and eating and of course postural positioning after meals. Also consider that a large percentage of digestion occurs with the help of gravity. If you were to eat launch and then hang upside down, you could imagine that digestion would be affected. Also consider how people sit after eating a quick lunch and then slouching in a chair back at the office. Digestion is a big part of how we feel throughout the day, and impairing the digestive process is obviously unwise.

You can see that the concept of postural analysis and the practice of postural therapy is a holistic medical idea. Postural alignment can invariably affect how we feel on the whole both in well-being and in illness. This is why I feel so strongly about the subject and a concept of postural therapy and correct postural awareness. There are very few subjects I am aware of that have a greater overall effect on general health. The insidious part of this subject is how nagging ailments can become potentially major health threats all leading back to a simple correctable postural problem. In its most basic form, this is very simple stuff. One of the first things we heard from our parents and grandparents was, "Stand up straight." Easily, some of the best advice ever given.

The Spiritual Journey Through Postural Therapy

Performing the exercises that are offered in this book and on the CD help release saratonin in the brain. The release of this chemical causes a calming affect and the following state of mind can be regarded as a spiritual journey. Once again this is subject matter that could be approached from an entire text full of concepts and case studies. Here again, our purposes are to merely approach the subject and idea that postural therapy can be a spiritual journey. First of all, the exercises themselves are healing and promote a renewed sense of well-being and energy. But the outcome or full reward of the exercises are an improved postural positioning and strengthening of postural muscles. This means that the muscles are taught to hold positions correctly, and this end in itself is the treasure at the end of the spiritual journey.

All spiritual journeys come with a warning, and that warning is that you should be emotionally prepared to surrender to these concepts. If your guard us up and your feelings are surrounded by brick walls, then nothing will be fulfilling. And that is essentially the warning. You must be willing to understand and believe that you will feel better and will experience improvement on several levels as you go through this program, and master the exercises as part of your lifestyle. If you are experiencing pain or feel that you have stagnated within a sport or other personal endeavors, you must be willing to let go of whatever is holding you back, and use this program to build a new bridge to personal improvement. Obviously there are many ways and many programs that can lead to an enhanced sense of well-being on many different levels. Some work well at certain periods throughout life and different programs will meet with more or less success. But here and now you are learning a specific program which in practice will not greatly change your lifestyle, but could greatly improve your life. In other words, you don't have to make any drastic changes in your life to systemati-cally bring this program into your life, but the outcome could be substantially beneficial. Simply put, practicing postural therapy gives back a lot of bang for the buck.

The Benefits of Sequential Focus

Throughout life many people but themselves through diets and exercise programs that are general in nature. They may decide to take up a walking program or some other exercise program such as swimming, jogging or a sport. And millions of people go on diets; some are quite specific and some are general conceptual diets such as low-fat, low cholesterol, or low-calorie diets. One of the key factors of postural therapy is the concept of sequential focus. The trick is to focus on one set of exercises that can fix a postural problem. Now this isn't always easy to figure out all by yourself which is why people practice postural therapy as a profession. But we can and will give you some direction as to sequences of exer-cises to focus on. You can think of it along these lines; do this set of exercises first for two weeks. Then do this set of exercises for the next two weeks. If your particular postural diagnosis has im-proved, then do the next set of exercises for the following two weeks. And then follow up with this final set of exercises to main-tain your maximum postural integrity.

Stop here and check out "Body Types & Exercises"

So the concept of postural analysis and the follow through with postural therapy is a sequential concept. There are very specific exercises designed for specific postural maladies. Each of these exercises are specifically timed and sequentially designed to im-prove specific physical attributes and muscle groups. This type of sequential focus is very different from the general idea of taking laps in the pool. General exercise programs and diets can be hard to follow because their pay off is more general in scope. Postural therapy techniques are very specific and the improvements sought as relief are also quite specific.

The exercises can be considered as a detailed set of instructions each designed to sequentially lead to the next step. Conceptually this differs greatly from most other weight and exercise programs. This program is more like putting together a toy that has specific instructions. These exercises are meant to the followed in a specific sequence which is different from most weight lifting programs or other types of exercise programs wherein the sequence is not necessarily important. Focusing on this sequence and the details helps give the mind greater concentration on the task at hand; which is to improve specific postural problems and the overall goal of greater health and vitality. To borrow and old phrase from a school-teacher, "inch by inch postural therapy is a sinch, yard by yard it can be hard."

One of the side benefits of focusing on details is that on a subconscious level your body will react. If you're thinking about the details of each exercise and sequentially preparing to move to the next exercise, your body will follow your mind like the cars of a train following the engine. The whole train will eventually get to its destination, but the engine has a very specific set of routines to accomplish the entire task.

The Science of Right Angles

There several principles and ideals which people have considered as a means for greater well-being. For example, if you smile all day, will you be happier? Well you certainly might appear so, but in reality you may not have any greater sense of well-being by smiling all day, and in fact you might find it irritating. Postural therapy is not metaphysical or even theoretical, it is simple good old-fashioned practical science. Your body was designed to function at right angles. Not all the joints, but the joints that we are concerned with were designed to function at right angles. If they're not positioned properly at right angles, they will not work as they were intended. People that perform at the highest physical peaks in the sports world typically have optimal postural alignment. You will note that there is usually a significant difference between an Olympic sprinter and a champion beer drinker. No doubt that both can perform their prospective tasks at championship levels, but their individual physical characteristics and overall physical health is usually quite different with regard to postural alignment.

Posture that is out of alignment is not an issue of perception but rather a stone cold reality. There are several issues regarding attitudes of human health that are perceptive rather than reality. In fact many symptoms are perceptions when the actual problem is a different reality. Pain resulting from compensation is just exactly such a reality and perception at the same time. The perception may be, for example, that you have a pain in your left shoulder. The reality might be that a misaligned hip is throwing of your balance and your left shoulder is compensating and being overworked and therefore soar and tender. Unfortunately, the medical community at large will look for the perceived problem which is pain in the shoulder and treat that symptom. But the cause of the pain, in this case, the misaligned hip, will again cause pain in that shoulder very soon.

Can We Ever Get Back to Basics?

Currently we're not a society of self reliant health experts. With thousands of volumes of books, videos and health programs available on the market, one might think that this society was clearly focused on personal health. More often the massive volume of information available serves to confuse us rather than assist us. Strangely, everybody has a new twist on how to become healthy with a machine that was designed millions of years ago. If the human body was in fact open to modifications in design prior to birth, notwithstanding hypothetical medical enhancements, certainly most people would be open to viable improvements. But the fact is, hypothetical medical enhancements are still hypothetical and experimental. They are not reality yet. So instead of wast-

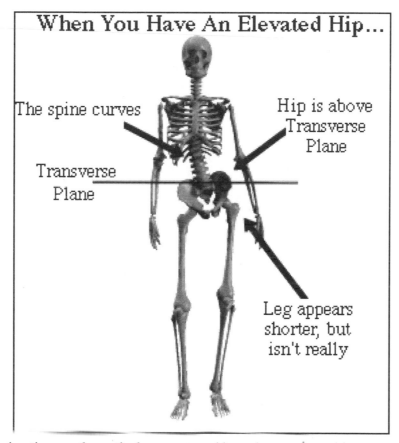

When You Have An Elevated Hip...

The spine curves

Hip is above Transverse Plane

Transverse Plane

Leg appears shorter, but isn't really

ing time on theoretical concepts and hypotheses why not try some good old-fashioned, back to the basics reality.

The human body is obviously designed with the capability of a seated position, but the human machine was built to move. All systems rely on movement to maintain optimal health. The only time the body is meant to be still is during periods of rest or healing from illness or injury. From there and after the body is meant to move, and that is **the basics**. It's really just that simple, if you move you stay healthy, if you stagnate, you become unhealthy. Sitting for hours a time is unhealthy, so you should get up and move around every hour if you have a job that requires a lot of "desk time." This is so basic it almost sounds meaningless and yet there is no more powerful advice or more meaningful information.

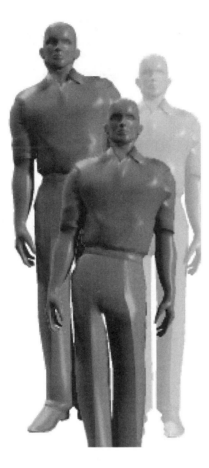

If you are someone who works at a job that requires a lot of time behind a desk, don't despair, because there are several things you can do to offset the lack of motion. But they do require some effort and exercise, but hopefully you'll find the exercises meaningful and sequentially beneficial. We're not talking about a change in lifestyle, but rather a prevention or maintenance program to assure that minimum but optimal movement is occurring. The type of exercise and movement is critical to the postural alignment needed for optimal health. This is why we have included very specific types of exercises designed exclusively for optimal postural alignment and maintenance.

A Look at the Postural Therapy Diagnosis Diagrams

The idea here is to stand in front of a mirror for a little self diagnosis. If you draw lines on the mirror you're likely to get a better idea of how you line up. Draw straight lines, obviously and make the cross sections 90 degree angles from the straight center line drawn in the middle. The following diagram should give you an idea of what to look for and how to draw it. You can use lipstick, or better yet an erasable marker just the same as those used on white boards. You should be able to wipe it off easily, but just a case test a little bit to make sure that you have no problem with erasable markers. Otherwise use lipstick, if you don't have any lipstick, by cheap lipstick, the quality won't matter.

Hopefully you have a little more weight that our model here. Starting with the feet, they should point straight. That is the original design and the way the feet and knees were designed. Certainly there are millions of people who have feet and knees aiming a little to the left or right or in some cases in opposite directions. For some people this will never pose a problem but they may find that some specific movement might be more difficult for them and as a result they will use other muscles to compensate for this situation. In other words, if your muscles are not lined up as originally designed, then you'll find a potential for compensation and musculature or pain problems can follow. One of the big problems comes with consistency regarding movement in a sport. You'll find that the vast majority of athletes that perform at the highest levels have their muscles and bones lined up in 90 degree angles as nature had originally designed and intended.

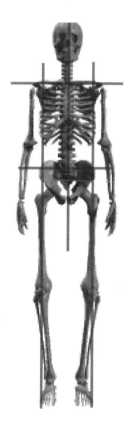

If your feet are pointing out like a duck or inward, sometimes called "pigeon towed," then your muscles must compensate for desired movement. It all makes perfect sense when you think of it this way; your body goes where you aim your feet. If you aim your feet to the left, you will turn to the left. If you aim your feet to the right, your body will move to the right. But what happens if your feet are pointing in opposite directions? The answer is, other muscles have to compensate to get your body moving in the direction you want to go. The problem is that these compensating muscles were not designed or intended for steering your body in one direction or another. But some people use them any way, and as a result, compensation occurs and more problems are potentially right around the corner.

For our purposes we'll leave the technical diagnostic terminology to the doctors because these particular situations are quite common and are very easy to understand. When feet point in, other muscles must compensate to help someone walk straight, and it's even more difficult to run straight. When feet point out a different set of muscles are used to perform the task of walking or running straight. Certainly it is possible to walk straight or run straight, but it requires the utilization of muscles that were not intended for this type of work. As our bodies have evolved over thousands of years it makes perfect sense that if you choose to use muscles incorrectly, there will be a price to pay at some point down the road.

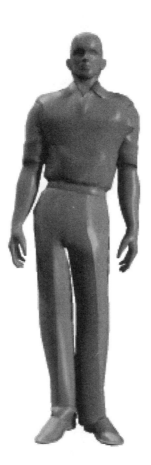

Now let's take a look at the hips. Like the knees or feet, the hips are meant to be on a straight horizontal line. Think of your hips as the top of a pendulum. Your legs swing forward and back, but if one side of your hip is a higher than the other, your legs will not swing consistently from the pendulum. As a result, other muscles will have to compensate for the fact that one leg is doing more work than the other. When your hips are not properly aligned, your whole body will compensate in many different ways. One of the most notable results is a loss of energy, and that can take a huge toll on any physical activity you might desire to participate in, including simple day-to-day movement.

An elevated hip can cause several unexpected problems.

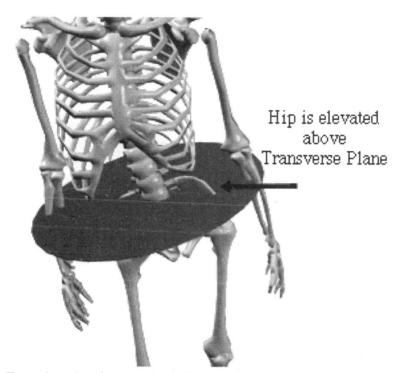

Hip is elevated
above
Transverse Plane

Try to imagine that your body is a car. But if your body is a car then what propels your body into motion? The answer is your hips. Your hips are the engine that drives and powers your motion. Without your hips you would have to rely on your arms for motion and quite simply, your arms were not designed to propel your body in motion. Your arms were designed to assist your body for tasks such as eating, working and so on. Interestingly, people don't often think about the importance of hips, and yet dysfunction in the hips and misalignment is one of the most serious issues that could ever confront a human body.

The hips actually work in a 360 X 360 degree environment. Obviously the hips don't work as simply as a two-dimensional pendulum. Your hips not only propel motion forward but also backward, side to side and up and down. Let's see if the engine a car can do that! Your hips are amazing and amazingly complex which is why it's so important that your posture supports your body in a healthful manner. When posture is bad, quite often it's the hips that take the hardest hit in the compensation department. Before too long your hips will ask other muscles to compensate for the problems that they have to deal with. The good news is that you can almost always correct postural maladies in the hips with a little information, some changes in habit and exercise.

Your hips can potentially tilt from the left to the right making it seem as though one leg is shorter than the other. Or the hips can tilt front to back causing abnormal curvatures in the back. Your hips can also be rotated in one direction or another. If you were standing up and a camera was pointing from the top of your head down toward your feet you might find that your hips have rotated slightly in one direction or another. Now you can see why we say that hips move in a 360X360 degree motion, and you can also see the amazing complexity of the engine that drives your body into motion.

Compensation typically occurs when the body asks superficial muscles to replace the work of intrinsic muscles. That means that there are muscles in any given area that will be moving differently and with a different type of load opposing their original design and purpose.

Quite often if someone is aware of the fact that they slouch or something about their posture is not quite correct, they will change their posture and positioning for diagnostic review. This is the absolute worst thing someone can do during diagnosis. The idea for a correct diagnosis is to stand in the same position that you would normally and with absolutely no conscious effort to correct your posture. If you have a problem that's posturally related and you're not truthful about your normal postural positioning and stance, then you have no means or legitimate measurement to compare for potential improvement. Some people naturally lean to one side or another. Other people might load most of their weight on one foot over the other. There are many conditions wherein people balance themselves or position themselves in one way or another which is posturally incorrect. Once they're made aware that their posture could be improved upon, then subconsciously they will alter their normal position during diagnosis. This is a very easy thing to do and you must try to maintain your normal position during diagnosis for comparative purposes later.

Here is a very simple analysis that should help you get a clear understanding of how gravity and your hips work together in concert. Think of a cross (see the illustration). The cross is six feet high with the horizontal intersection directly in the center of the vertical piece. Imagine that all of the pieces are square and plum. That means that the horizontal piece intersects the vertical piece at a perfect 90 degree angle. The cross can stand up on its own because it is perfectly balanced. Now what would happen if you shifted the horizontal crossmember a few inches to one side or the other? The answer is that the cross would tip over because it is out of balance. But there are other solutions. You could bevel the bottom base of the cross so that it is at an angle which compensates for the out posi-

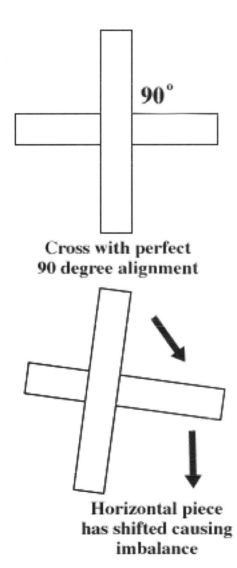

90°

**Cross with perfect
90 degree alignment**

**Horizontal piece
has shifted causing
imbalance**

tion horizontal cross member. Or you could tilt the top piece of the cross so it's weight would compensate for the out of position horizontal cross member.

If you're hips are out of alignment to the point where you sense a lack of balance, you either compensate or fall over, just like the cross. If the cross is out of alignment it will fall over unless the out of balance piece is compensated for in one way or another. Your body works just the same and will find ways to compensate so it can function normally without interruption. But as the body utilizes superficial muscles for compensation, the

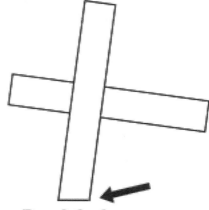

**Bevel the base
to maintain balance
1st Compensation...**

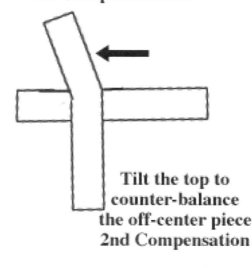

**Tilt the top to
counter-balance
the off-center piece
2nd Compensation**

muscles intended for such specific movement will atrophy creating a whole new set of problems. In essence, a cycle of problems will begin when muscular compensation starts.

Interesting Realizations

There are many people who are diagnosed with having one leg shorter than the other, but this specific condition is actually very rare. The vast majority of the situations related to the hip area is that the hip has shifted up or down on one side. In reality the legs are the same length. The shifting gives the appearance and symptomatic condition of having one leg shorter than the other. People with such a condition are often prescribed special shoes with a height lifter built in. The exercise category for an elevated hip problem is called a Transverse Plane exercise. These are exercises that are designed to alleviate problems in the Transverse Plane. The Transverse Plane is the horizontal plain that our bones line up with when positioned correctly. When bones protrude through the transverse plain compensation will occur because natural balance will become an issue. Take a look at our skeleton friend who has an elevated hip.

When a building is constructed its vertical walls are built perpendicular to gravity. Meaning that the walls are designed to be constructed at 90 degree angles to gravity to create the greatest possible strength. Our bodies were built the same way and were meant to be aligned 90 degrees perpendicular to gravity. When a building is out of alignment, its structural integrity is at risk, and the same holds true with our body. The foundation of our body could be considered the hips, which is why the concepts of postural therapy place so much importance on the hips.

The Wrong Kind of Exercise Is Still Wrong

Staying with our hips as our foundation analogy, think of a building project. Let's say that you want to build an incredibly strong house. You get the best materials such as commercial brick. You reinforce it with steel to make it even stronger. You use only the finest most expensive cements to keep your bricks and steel in place for centuries. Then you take this incredible building and set it on top of a Balsa Wood foundation. Eventually the foundation will collapse and the house in all its strength and glory will fall over.

Staying in a seated position all day has a similar effect as building a rock solid house on a poor foundation. Strengthening the chest shoulders and arms does nothing to improve the condition of the most important aspect of the human body, the hips. Staying in a seated position keeps the arms and shoulders in action but takes the motion engine into neutral. In a neutral position the hips will eventually atrophy and lose the ability to maneuver the body as required, and places the body in eminent danger regarding sudden movement such as falls or collisions. The name of the game is to keep the hips moving and strong. In concept it's very simple, but in practice it requires some diligence and a conscious effort to exercise correctly.

Consider the Right Concept

Special equipment, shoes and ergonomic furniture may help relieve the symptoms but they will not correct the problem. If a hip is misaligned there are specific exercises that will help reposition it and also help the correct muscles to hold it in place permanently. This is the right concept and the right approach to handling an alignment problem. The answer is not to mask symptoms or heal symptoms, but to correct the problem that caused the symptoms. Virtually all postural alignment conditions can be corrected with be right type of exercise in the correct sequence. It's actually a very basic and simple premise. For those who would like a more complicated and technical procedure to correct postural problems we recommend the medical section at your local library. But if you're honestly concerned with real world answers based on the simple concepts of 90 degree alignment against the constant force of gravity, postural therapy is the answer.

Section 2.
Introduction to Body Types and Exercises

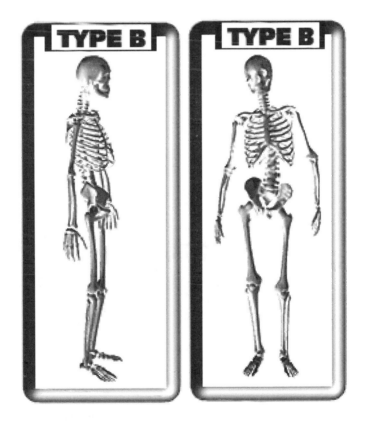

Body types can be called Type 1 or A, Type 2 or B and Type 3 or C. The numbers and letters are interchangeable. The most important thing to remember is that you need to identify which body type you most closely resemble.

It seems reasonable to consider that there might be an endless variety of body types but oddly, most people fall into one of four categories. The last category, (ideal posture) really isn't even a category but we can't call it normal either, because ideal postural alignment is not normal in most adults. Most people have a type of postural malady that is similar to one of the three body types we have listed here. Certainly any one individual will have a little more or less tweaking to do, to perfectly match the body types. Overall these are the types of bodies that seem to be walking into Symmetry The Pain Relief Clinic, in San Diego most often.

When you are performing your own Self-Diagnosis, look for the types of maladies that you see for the body type graphics that we have presented for you. You might not necessarily be one type or another, but try to estimate as closely as possible which body type you most likely resemble.

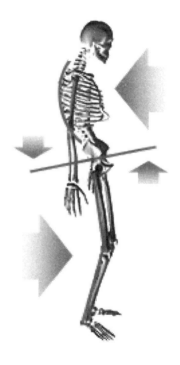

We will start with a very common postural condition, we call, body type A, illustrated on the next page. Now if you happen to be one of those rare people that seem to have good postural alignment all and all, look for the small things such as knees, feet and shoulder directions. Above all, think prevention. Just because you've not developed a postural problem yet, does not mean that you won't. We're all living in an automated lifestyle and as such we are prone to the disposition for postural problems. It is imminent that anyone who lives a modern lifestyle of today, will find themselves fighting pains associated with the lack of proper motion in the fu-

The forces of gravity and time can eventually break down posture.

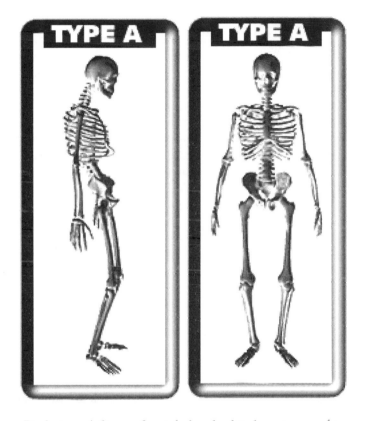

ture. Body type A from a frontal view looks almost normal to most people. That's the interesting thing, that poor posture looks normal because so many people have it. Note from the frontal position the feet and knees are pointing outward which is less than ideal and causes muscular strains in the lower back and loss of energy in the back of legs and hips. One tell-tail sign of rounded shoulders from the frontal view, is that you can see the backs of the hands, because the arms and forearms are rolled inward. But the real story is told from the side view. If you're on the computer now, click on the side view and see what the body types look like from the side.

From the side you can see that body type A is in big trouble. The knees are in front of the shoulders, the hips are in front of the shoulders, and the arms are hanging behind the hips. The head is leaning forward and from here on the news gets worse. The feet and

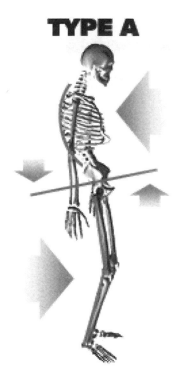

TYPE A

ankles are subject to soreness and injury; the back is curved which leads to headaches, jaw pain, neck pain and drooping shoulders. Because the back is curved or hunched, there is pressure placed on the chest and lungs which decreases the capacity for deep breathing. As a result, less oxygen is taken into the lungs and utilized for replenishment. This hunched position also puts a strain on the digestive system which is compressed as well. Type A bodies are also associated with depression and a lack of self esteem, because hunched over people look tired and sad.

Body type B, illustrated on the following page, is also very common and is quickly evidenced by someone who stands with one foot in front of the other somewhat similar to the frontal view of the graphic for type B. The condition for type B is known as elevation. Generally one side of the hip is higher than the other which leads to a misalignment in the shoulders. To compensate for the misalignment the spine typically curves in the opposite direction of the elevated hip to keep the body as level as possible. The feet and legs must adjust for this difference in apparent length, because with an elevated hip your body adjusts as though one leg is longer than the other. As you can imagine this condition throws off all types of movement, and greatly hampers concise actions in sports.

For example if you were to take golf lessons, the golf instructor would not likely take into consideration postural characterizations. Therefore you would be taught to swing a club as though your body was properly aligned. As such, you would never have a chance

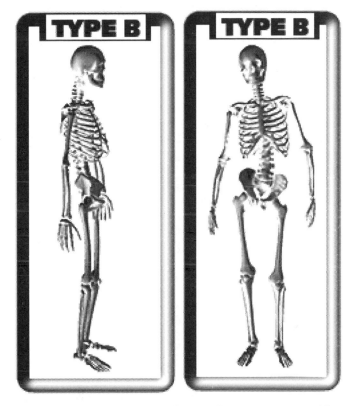

at a consistent swing because that golf pro wasn't teaching you how to swing a club based on your postural malady. The truth is, you can miss a lot when your postural structure is out of alignment. There might be several things that you could be good at, but will have trouble mastering because your body will not allow you to work with the consistency required to master the task or sport.

People with B type bodies are often diagnosed with one leg shorter than the other and fitted with special lifter shoes. This serves to only make the problem worse. People whose shoulders are elevated are often instructed to sit in special chairs and even place a book under one hip to help with realignment. Type B's suffer from headaches and back aches and often place weight incorrectly throughout their daily activities. The good news is that hip elevation problems are typical, readily understood by postural therapists and have specific and easy exercises to correct the problem and keep it away.

Body type C is another combination of postural problems. From the front view you'll note that the feet and knees are rotated outward. The shoulders have a tendency to elevate to the stronger more dominant side. Left-handed people will be slightly elevated to the left side and right-handed people will have a shoulder eleva-

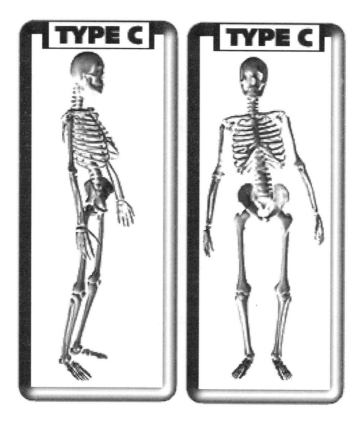

tion for the right side. From the hips up the body will tend to lean a little bit toward the weaker side. The reason for all of this is decreased strength in the hip musculature which has allowed the body to lean with an emphasis on side of domination, right or left. Since the hips shift forward, there is a tendency toward sway back and the natural "S" curve in the back becomes more of a "C" curve.

The head must lean forward to help compensate for weight distribution issues from the "Sway Back." Now you can understand the concepts and requirements for compensation. When the body is out of alignment, muscles and bones must compensate in various ways to assure that your body will be able to maintain balance for daily activities. People with sway back often have terrible back aches and sense pain from long walks and running. The head leaning forward causes a stretching motion on the back shoulder muscles and spine leading to fatigue, jaw strain and headaches. Eventually a sway back condition will lead to compression in the lower back as the situation precipitates shortened back muscles in the lower back. The shortened back muscles only complicate the matter and lower spinal disc problems could occur in later years. Type C's are easy to fix, and you will find the the exercises are relaxing and stimulating at the same time. A reverse "C" curve in the back is nothing to ignore, but it is fairly easy to remedy over a relatively short period of time.

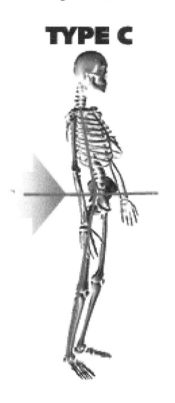

TYPE C

In the previous pages we have shown illustrations of ideal posture. The key thing to remember is that optimal performance does not necessarily follow ideal posture. Flexibility, range of motion, strength and endurance all must be considered as factors in optimal performance. So if you feel that you are one of the lucky ones with ideal, or nearly ideal posture, don't forget to work on other aspects of your physical condition. Strive to improve flexibility and hip strength. Work on the exercises in the exercise section of the book and CD-ROM that seem the most challenging. Most importantly, never take ideal posture for granted, because one day something may happen that could cause the beginning of muscular compensations.

Here is a list of professions and potential body types that often occur after a number of years working in one of the following professions.

Accountant, Body Type C
Actor/Actress, Body Type B
Architect, Body Type A
Attorney, Body Type A
Chiropractic, Body Type A
Computer Programmer/Analyst, Body Type A
Dancer, Body Type A
Dentist, Body Type A
Engineer, Body Type B
Executive, Body Type C
Firefighter, Body Type C
Flight Attendant, Body Type B
Golfer, Body Type C
Housewife, Body Type B
Journalist, Body Type A
Nurse, Body Type B
Optometrist, Body Type A
Personal Assistant, Body Type B
Photographer, Body Type A
Physical Therapist, Body Type B
Physician, Body Type A
Pilot, Body Type A
Police Officer, Body Type A
Professional Athlete, Body Type C
Professor/Teacher, Body Type B
Real Estate Agent, Body Type B
Salesperson, Body Type A
Tradesman, Body Type C
Writer/Author, Body Type A

Body Type A and Associated Exercises

Exercise Group 1

Static Floor — 5: 00 (Do for Five Minutes)
Shin Burners (Static Floor) — 2 Sets of 30 Repetitions, 1 Set of 20

Hip Abduction/Adduction — 2 Sets of 30 Repetitions
Extended Floor Position (Elbows) — (Do for Two Minutes)
Piriformis Stretch (Floor) — One Minute per Side
Piriformis Stretch (Crossover) — One Minute per Side
Pelvic Tilts — 15 Repetitions
Lying Groin Stretch — (Do for Two Minutes)
Floor Press (In Lying Growing Stretch Position) — 30 Repetitions
Extended Floor Position — (Do for Two Minutes)

Exercise Group 2

Static Floor — (Do for Five Minutes)
Inverted Wall — (Do for Two Minutes)
Arm Pullovers (Inverted Wall) — 20 Repetitions
Hip Adduction (Sitting) — Three Sets of 20 Repetitions
Shoulder Shrugs (Sitting) — Two Sets of 20 Repetitions
Kneeling Ankle Press (Block) — 45 Repetitions
Extended Ankle Abduction — 45 Repetitions
Standing Overhead Reach — (Do for One Minute)

Exercise Group 3

Gluteal Squeezes — 60 Repetitions
Hip Abduction (Hooklying) — 45 Repetitions
Hip Adduction (Hooklying) — 45 Repetitions
Hip Adduction (Sitting) — Three Sets of 20 Repetitions
Gravity Drop — (Do for 3 Minutes)
Floor Press (Hooklying) — 30 Repetitions
Piriformis Stretch (Wall) — One Minute per Side
Shin Burners (Wall) — 2 Sets of 30 Repetitions, 1 Set of 20
Extended Floor Position — (Do for Two Minutes)
Wall Set — (Do for One Minute)

Exercise group 4

Static Floor — (Do for Five Minutes)
Floor Press (In Static Floor Position) — 30 Repetitions
Arm Pullovers (In Static Floor Position) — 20 Repetitions
Lying Groin Stretch — (Do for Two Minutes)
Abdominal Crunches (Lying Groin Stretch) — 2 Sets of 20 Rep-
etitions

Piriformis Stretch (Crossover) — One Minute per Side
Cats and Dogs — 10 Repetitions
Hip Adduction (Hooklying) — 45 Repetitions
Sitting Knee Raises (Block) — 3 Sets of 20 Repetitions
Shoulder Rotations (Kneeling) — 20 Repetitions
Rolls (Settle) — Do for Five Minutes

Body Type B and Associated Exercises

Exercise Group 1

Static Floor — (Do for Five Minutes)
Floor Press (Static Floor) — 30 Repetitions
Hip Abduction (Static Floor) — 3 Sets of 20 Repetitions
Prone Blocked Floor — (Do for Six Minutes)
Hip Abduction/Adduction — 2 Sets of 30 Repetitions
Piriformis Stretch (Wall) — One Minute per Side
Pelvic Tilts — 10 Repetitions
Hip Abduction (Static) — (Do for Three Minutes)
Wall Set — (Do for Two Minutes)

Exercise Group 2

Static Floor — (Do for Five Minutes)
Overhead Press — 30 Repetitions
Extended Ankle Press (Block) — 45 Repetitions
Cats and Dogs — 45 Repetitions
Piriformis Stretch (Crossover) — One Minute per Side
Kneeling Overhead Reach — (Do for One Minute)
Rolls Heel/Toe (Strap) — Two Sets of 30 Repetitions
Rolls (Settle) — (Do for Five Minutes)
Wall Sit — (Do for Two Minutes)

Exercise Group 3

Static Floor — (Do for Five Minutes)
Floor Clock — Three Sets of One Minute Each
Abdominal Crunches (Wall) — Two Sets of 20 Repetitions
Buddha's Pose — (Do for One Minute)
Overhead Extension (in Buddha's Pose) — (Do for One Minute)
Sitting Torso Twist — (Do for One Minute)
Cats and Dogs — 10 Repetitions

Lying Hip Flex or Stretch — Two Minutes per Leg
Downward Dog — (Do for One Minute)

Exercise Group 4

Static Floor — (Do for Five Minutes)
Shin Burners — Two Sets of 40, One Set of 20
Prone Opposite Glides — Five Repetitions of 10 Seconds Each
Crunches (Lying Groin Stretch) — Two Sets of 25 Repetitions
Lower Spinal Floor Twist — Two Minutes per Side
Cats and Dogs — 10 Repetitions
Hip Adduction (Sitting) — Three Sets of 20 Repetitions
Pec Stretch — Three Sets of 10 Repetitions
Overhead Extension (Sitting) — (Do for One Minute)
Squat — (Do for One Minute)

Body Type C and Associated Exercises

Exercise Group 1

Static Floor — (Do for Five Minutes)
Abdominal Crunches (Static Floor) — Two Sets of 25 Repetitions
Prone Blocked Floor — (Do for Six Minutes)
Piriformis and Stretch (Wall) — One Minute per Side
Hip Abduction (Static Floor) — 45 Repetitions
Piriformis Stretch (Crossover) — One Minute per Side
Cats and Dogs — 10 Repetitions
Straight Arm Rotations (Kneeling) — Two Sets of 30 Repetitions
Shoulder Rotations — 20 Repetitions
Psoas Stretch (Progressive) — Keep Level for Three Minutes
Wall Set — (Do for Two Minutes)

Exercise Group 2

Static Floor — (Do for Five Minutes)
Prone Ankle Press — 45 Repetitions
Striking Cobra — 45 Repetitions
Floor Clock — One Minute per Side
Piriformis Stretch (Crossover) — One Minute per Side
Piriformis Stretch (Floor) — One Minute per Side
Cats and Dogs — 10 Repetitions

Overhead Extension (Buddha's Pose) — (Do for One Minute)
Kneeling Overhead Stretch (Crossed) —(Do for One Minute)
Wall Sit —(Do for Two Minutes)

Exercise Group 3

Static Floor — (Do for Five Minutes)
Prone Blocked Floor — (Do for Five Minutes)
Arm Pullovers (Static Floor) — 30 Repetitions
Inverted Wall — (Do for Five Minutes)
Arm Pullovers (Inverted Wall) — 30 Repetitions
Lower Spinal Floor Twist — Two Minutes per Side
Cats and Dogs — 10 Repetitions
Standing Overhead Stretch —(Do for One Minute)
Wall Sit — (Do for Two Minutes)

Exercise Group 4

Static Floor — (Do for Five Minutes)
Sitting Knee Sequence — One Minute per Side
Extended Ankle Abduction — 45 Repetitions
Sitting Torso Twist — (Do for One Minute)
Cats and Dogs — 10 Repetitions
Wall Sit — (Do for Two Minutes)
Gravity Drop (Wall) — Do for Six Minutes
Shoulder Rotations (Gravity Drop) — 30 Repetitions

Here are some of the more common pain groups and some exercises that can help remedy them.

Headaches /T. M. J./ Neck Pain

1. Extended Floor Position — Two Minutes
2. Piriformis Stretch (Crossover) — One Minute
3. Pelvic Tilts — 10 Repetitions
4. Extended Floor Position — Two Minutes
5. Wall Sit — One Minute
6. Rolls (Settle) — Ten Minutes

Shoulder/Mid Back Pain

1. Static Floor — Five Minutes
2. Arm Pullovers — 30 Repetitions
3. Prone Blocked Floor — Five Minutes
4. Cats and Dogs — 10 Repetitions
5. Shoulder Rotations (Standing) — Two Sets of 20 Repetitions
6. Extended Floor Position — Two Minutes

Low Back Pain/Strain

1. Static Floor — Five Minutes
2. Hip Abduction/Adduction — Two Sets of 30 Repetitions
3. Hip Abduction (Hooklying) — 45 Repetitions
4. Abdominal Crunches (Wall) — Two Sets of 25 Repetitions
5. Piriformis Stretch (Crossover) — One Minute per Side
6. Cats and Dogs — 10 Repetitions
7. Wall Sit — Two Minutes

Hip Pain, Gluteal Pain

1. Static Floor — Five Minutes
2. Piriformis Stretch (Floor) — One Minute per Side
3. Hip Adduction (Hooklying) — 45 Repetitions
4. Piriformis Stretch (Wall) — One Minute per Side
5. Inverted Wall — Two Minutes
6. Arm Pullovers (Static Floor) — 30 Repetitions
7. Wall Set — Two Minutes

Knee Pain

1. Hip Adduction (Sitting) — Three Sets of 20 Repetitions
2. Straight Arm Rotations (Sitting) — 40 Repetitions
3. Floor Clock — One Minute per Side
4. Hip Adduction (Hooklying) — 45 Repetitions
5. Overhead Press (Hooklying) — 45 Repetitions
6. Standing Overhead Reach — One Minute

Ankle/Foot Pain

1. Static Floor — Five Minutes
2. Shin Burners (In Static Floor) — Two Sets of 40, One Set of 20

3. Heel/Toe (Strap) — Two Sets of 30 Repetitions
4. Piriformis Stretch (Floor) — One Minute per Side
5. Cats and Dogs — 10 Repetitions
6. Hip Abduction (Static) — Three Minutes
7. Wall Sit — Two Minutes

Elbow/Wrist Pain...Tennis Elbow/Carpal Tunnel

1. Shoulder Rotations (Standing) — 30 Repetitions
2. Wall Push — One Minute
3. Extended Floor Position — Two Minutes
4. Cats and Dogs — 10 Repetitions
5. Sitting Torso Twist — One Minute per Side
6. Cats and Dogs — 10 Repetitions
7. Overhead Extension (Standing) — One Minute

Section 3. The Exercises Listed Alphabetically

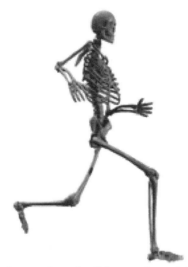

There are a lot of exercises in this section. Most of them are listed here for reference or as companions to some of the more basic exercises. If you ever find yourself working directly with a postual therapist, such as the Symmetry Clinic, in Del Mar California, then you will have this list ready to go. Feel free to experiment with any of these exercises AFTER you have completed your recommended program. In other words, don't skip around, do the exercises associated with your body type first, and complete your program. Once you are back on track, then feel free to maintain your optimal posture with some other exercises for added variety.

Abdominal Crunches (Static Floor)

1

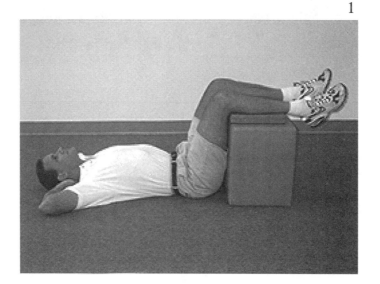

In Static Floor position clasp hands behind head with elbows touching the floor. While looking back, raise elbows, shoulders and head off floor using abdominal muscles. Then return to starting position.

2

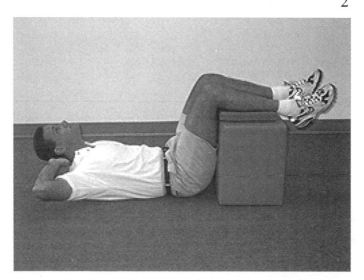

Abdominal Crunches (Wall)

1

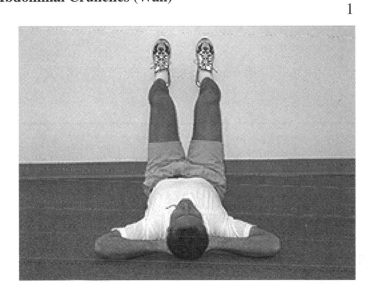

On back with knees and hips bent at 90 degree, place feet hip-width and straight on wall. While looking back raise elbows, shoulders and head off floor using abdominal muscles. Then return to starting position with elbows, shoulders and head touching floor.

2

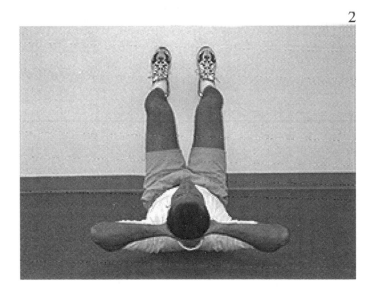

Abdominal Squeezes(Static Floor

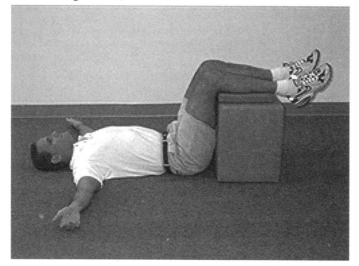

In Static Floor position inhale while pushing stomach up; breathe out by letting stomach fall. Upon end of exhalation tighten abdominal muscles and hold for one second and release.

Active Hurdle Stretch

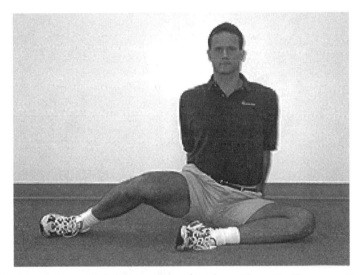

Sitting on floor with hips square, bend one knee in front on floor with foot in. Bend the other knee 90 degrees placing foot out to side. Prop hands behind for minor support, and roll hips forward as much as possible while trying to maintain even pressure on buttocks on floor. Press and release knee into pillow; then lift and lower knee maintaining the above position. Then switch leg position. RELAX STOMACH.

Ankle/Knee Press (No Lift)

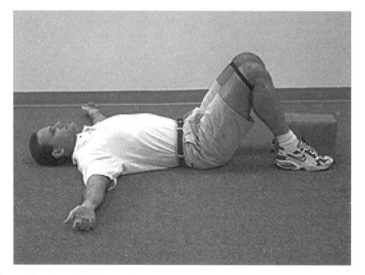

Lie on back with knees bent and feet flat on floor (hip-width). Simultaneously, press out on strap at knees and in on 6" block between feet. Make sure feet stay flat on floor and squeeze pillow with inside of heel and toes. Relax stomach and shoulders throughout exercise.

Ankle/Knee Opposite (No Lift)

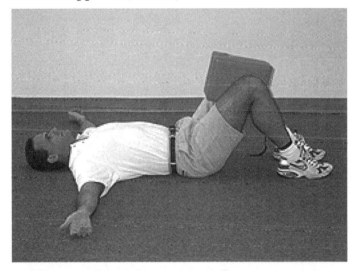

Place strap around ankles and knees. Simultaneously, press and release pillow at knees and strap at ankles keeping feet flat on floor. Relax stomach and shoulders throughout exercise.

Ankle/Knee Opposite Press

1

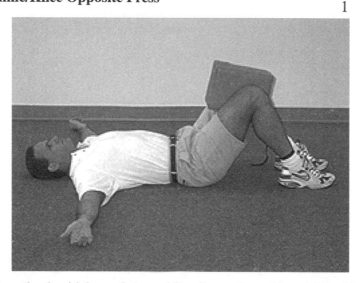

Lie on back with knees bent and feet flat on floor (hip-width). Place 7"pillow between knees and strap around ankles. While maintaining constant pressure out on strap and in on block, pull knees towards chest, lifting feet 3-4" off floor. Keep knees bent at 90 degrees while focusing. Lift from hips and not stomach. Relax shoulders and breathe!

2

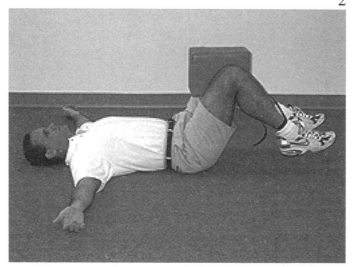

Ankle/Knee Press

1

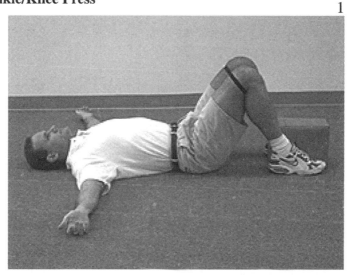

Lie on back with knees bent and feet flat on floor (hip-width). Place strap around knees and 6" block between feet. While maintaining constant pressure out on strap and in on block, pull knees towards chest, lifting feet 3-4" off floor. Keep knees bent at 90 degrees. While focusing, lift from hips and not stomach. Relax shoulders and breathe!

2

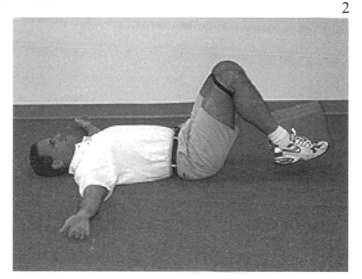

Arm Glides (Gravity Drop)

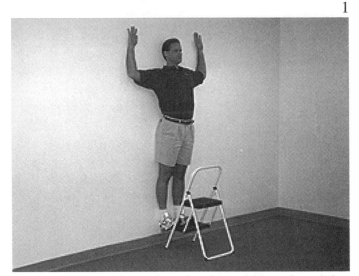

In Gravity Drop position, place feet hip width and straight with heels almost touching wall. Place upper arms directly out to side with elbows bent at 90 degrees so that back of forearms and hands are touching the wall. With legs straight and stomach relaxed, slowly glide arms above head while maintaining 90 degree angle until hands touch. Then return to starting position. Make Sure that arms and hands remain on the wall throughout motion. Inhale on the way up.

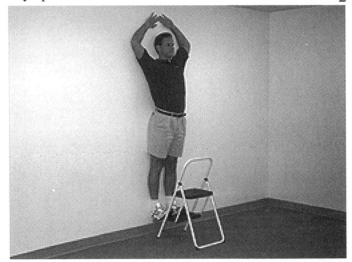

Arm Glides (Standing)

1

Standing against wall, place feet hip width and straight with heels touching wall. Place upper arms directly out to side with elbows bent at 90 degrees so that back of forearms and hands are touching the wall. With legs straight and stomach relaxed, slowly glide arms above head while maintaining 90 degree angle until hands touch, then return to starting position.. Make sure that arms and hands remain on the wall throughout motion. Inhale on the way up.

2

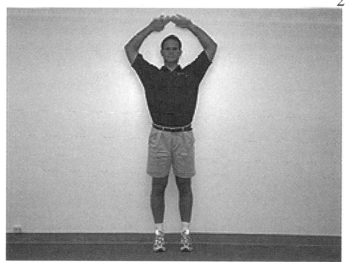

Arm Glides (Wall Sit) Sitting against wall with buttocks as close to wall as possible, keep legs straight out and hip width. Pull toes back: tighten quads with knees pointed to ceiling; push stomach out and keep relaxed. Place back of arms on wall with elbows bent at 90 degrees. While pushing arms into wall, slowly glide arms above head keeping elbows bent at 90 degree until hands touch. Return arms to starting position and repeat. Make sure elbows and back of hands remain touching wall throughout motion.

Arm Pullovers (Hooklying)   1

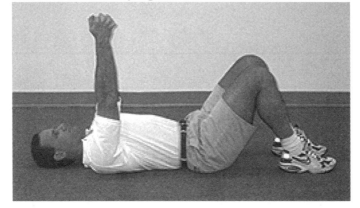

On back with knees bent, feet hip width and straight, clasp hands together with arms straight, pointed to ceiling, and shoulders settled to floor. Slowly reach hands towards floor overhead keeping arms straight, elbows locked and palms together. Only lower arms as far as you can without bending elbows, then return to starting position and repeat. Inhale when reaching to floor, allowing back to arch and stomach to relax.

2

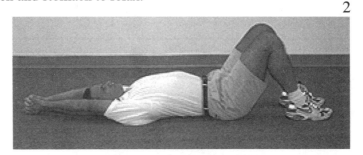

Arm Pullovers (Inverted Wall) 1

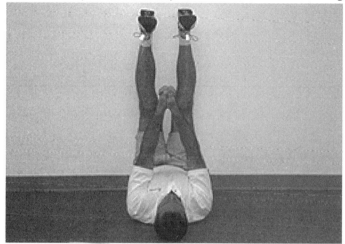

Lie on back with legs straight up on wall, feet hip width apart. With quads tight, position body away from wall, if necessary, so that tail bone rests on floor. Keep knees pointed away from wall and toes flexed back. Clasp hands together with arms straight, pointed to ceiling, and shoulders settled to floor. Slowly reach hands towards floor overhead keeping arms straight, elbows locked and palms together. Only lower arms as far as you can without bending elbows, then return to starting position and repeat. Inhale when reaching to floor, allowing back to arch and stomach to relax. 2

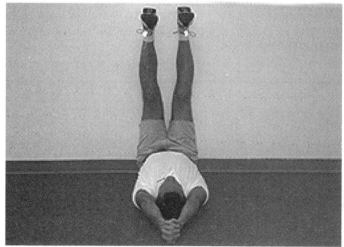

Arm Pullovers (Lying Groin Stretch)

On back with knees bent, place feet together and allow knees to separate until bottom of soles come together. Clasp hands together with arms straight, pointed to ceiling, and shoulders settled to floor. Slowly reach hands towards floor overhead keeping arms straight, elbows locked and palms together. Only lower arms as far as you can without bending elbows. Then return to starting position and repeat. Inhale when reaching to floor, allowing back to arch and stomach to relax.

Arm Pullovers (Static Floor)

1

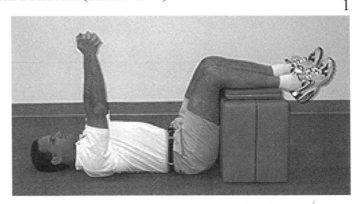

With legs propped on block, knees bent at 90 degrees, clasp hands together with arms straight, pointed to ceiling, and shoulders settled to floor. Slowly reach hands towards floor overhead keeping arms straight, elbows locked and palms together. Only lower arms as far as you can without bending elbows, then return to starting position and repeat. Inhale when reaching to floor, allowing back to arch and stomach to relax.

2

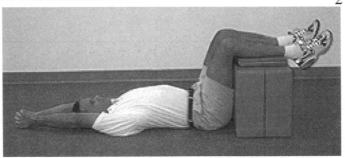

Blanket Stretch

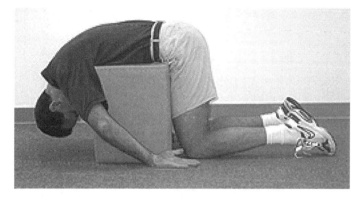

Drape body over 18"-high block or chair. Keep upper body re-laxed letting arms, shoulders and head fall to the floor. BREATHE through diaphragm and feel stretch in lower back.

Buddha's Pose

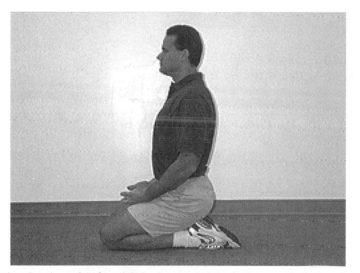

Sitting back on heels with knees together, induce arch in low back by rolling hips forward and not by leaning back. Hold position for allotted time while relaxing shoulders and stomach.

Buddha's Squat

1

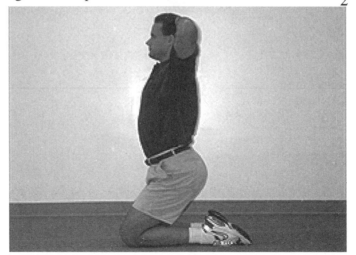

Sitting back on heels with knees together, induce arch in lower back by rolling hips forward and not by leaning back. Interlace hands behind head pulling elbows back, and lift body off heals maintaining arch in low back. Lift up only as high as arch can be maintained. Then return to starting position. Do not lean forward or back throughout motion, and repeat for allotted repetitions. Feel in thighs and keep stomach relaxed.

2

Buddha's Twist

Sitting back on heels with knees together, induce arch in low back by rolling hips forward and not by leaning back. Interlace hands behind head and pull elbows back. While keeping arch in low back and elbows pulled back, slowly twist upper torso to one side without moving hips and tightening stomach. Hold position for allotted time, switch to the other side and hold. Then return to the middle and hold for remainder of time allotted.

Carpet Glides (Hook Lying)

1

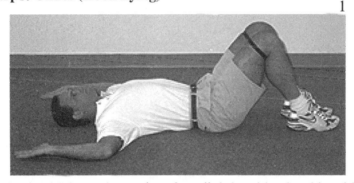

On back with knees bent, place feet slightly wider than hip width. Bring knees together and pull strap tight. Maintaining constant pressure out on strap, bend elbows at 90 degrees placing arms and back of hands on floor. Maintaining a 90 degree angle, slowly raise arms overhead until hands touch keeping elbows, forearms and hands slightly pressed into floor. Return to starting position and repeat for allotted number of repetitions. Be sure to inhale and allow back to arch as you reach arms overhead.

2

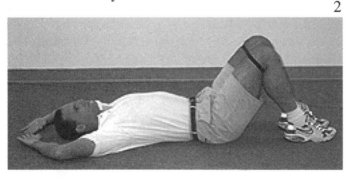

Carpet Glides (Inverted Wall)   1

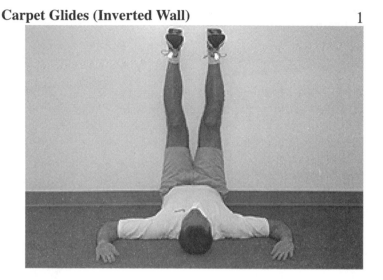

Lie on back with legs straight up on wall, feet hip width apart.
With quads tight position body away from wall, if necessary, so
that tail bone rests on floor. Keeping knees pointed away from
wall and toes flexed back, bend elbows at 90 degrees placing arms
and back of hands on floor. Maintaining a 90 degree angle, slowly
raise arms overhead until hands touch keeping elbows, forearms
and hands slightly pressed into floor. Return to starting position
and repeat for allotted number of repetitions. Be sure to inhale and
allow back to arch as you reach arms overhead.   2

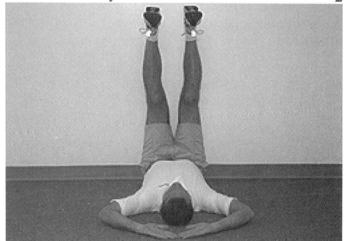

Carpet Glides (Static Floor)

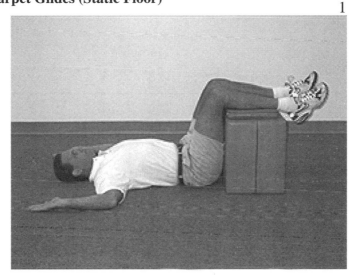

1

With legs propped on block, knees bent at 90 degrees, bend elbows at 90 degrees placing arms and back of hands on floor. Maintaining a 90 degree angle, slowly raise arms overhead until hands touch keeping elbows, forearms and hands slightly pressed into floor. Return to starting position and repeat for allotted number of repetitions. Be sure to inhale and allow back to arch as you reach arms overhead.

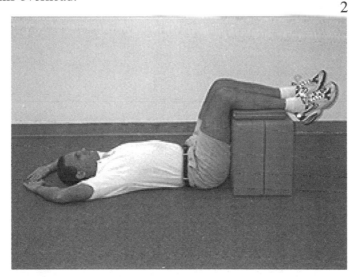

2

Cats and Dogs

1

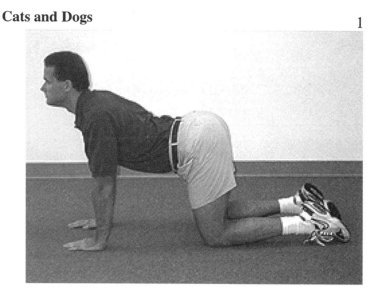

Start with hands and knees hip width apart and perpendicular to the floor. Pull chin to chest while pushing low back to ceiling. Then look up to ceiling and allow back to sway and shoulder blades to pull back and together. Keep a constant, smooth motion not allowing your body to move forward or backwards.

2

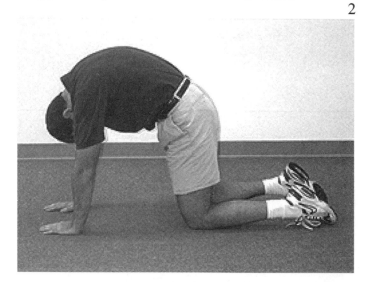

Cervical Stretch

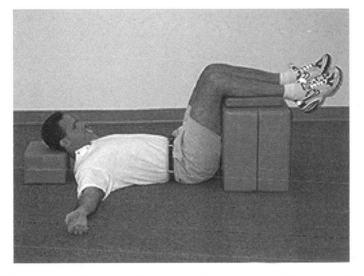

While in static floor postition,, head is resting on 6" block. Block must be placed on a flat surface behind head. Let head settle into chest and breathe.

Cobra (On Elbows)

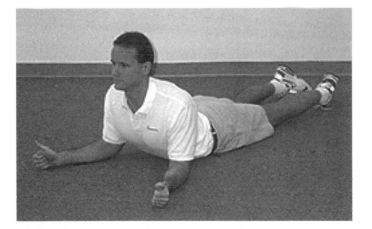

In prone position, prop elbows under shoulders and pull forearms apart while keeping hands on floor, thumbs pointing to ceiling. Allow feet to pigeon-toe by relaxing abdominals and glutes. Feel in lower back.

Cobra (On Hands)

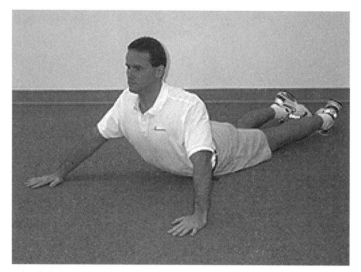

In prone position with feet pigeon-toed, place hands out to side and straighten arms out allowing torso to raise off the floor. Keeping hips on floor, pull shoulder blades back and together. Be careful not to shrug shoulders. Relax stomach and glutes and feel in lower back.

Core Abs

Position 1: On back with legs straight, prop elbows under shoulder, pull toes back and lift pelvis off floor and hold. Position 2: Lying on side prop elbow underneath shoulder with forearm and hand on floor. Keeping body straight, place feet together and lift hips off floor. Keep opposite arm at your side allowing shoulder blades to squeeze together. Position 3: Same as 2nd position-opposite side. Position 4: Lying on stomach, prop elbows under shoulders with forearms and hands on floor. Curl toes under keeping feet hip-width, tighten quads and lift hips off floor. Let shoulder blades collapse together while pushing hips to ceiling. Hold for allotted amount of time.

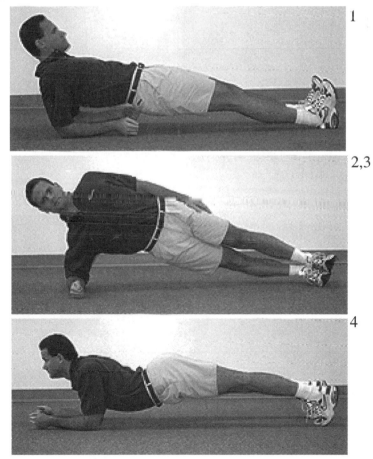

1

2,3

4

Crunches (Lying Groin Stretch)

1

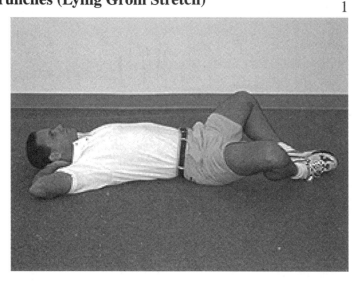

On back with knees bent, place feet together and allow knees to separate until bottom of soles come together. While looking back, raise elbows, shoulders and head off floor using abdominal muscles. Then return to starting position with elbows, shoulders and head touching floor.

2

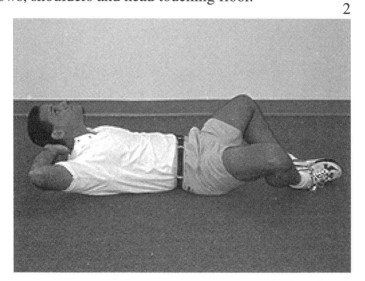

Decline Wall Sit

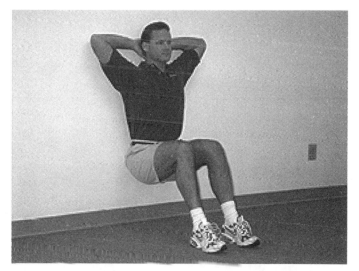

With low back against wall, slowly walk feet out away from wall. Keeping feet hip width and pointing straight ahead, slide down wall until knees are below 90 degrees making sure ankles are in front of knees. Place hands on head keeping elbows back and allow back to arch by lifting toes off floor and stomach relaxed. Feel in thighs and hip flexors.

Downward Dog

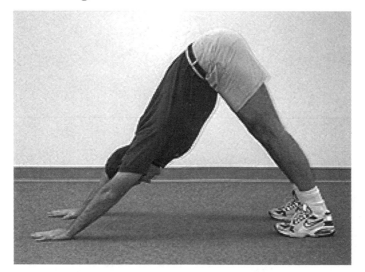

Start with hands and knees hip width apart and perpendicular to the floor. Curling toes under, lift knees off floor by tightening quads and maintaining arch in low back. Without moving hands or feet, push head and chest through arms towards knees while still maintaining arch in low back and quad tight. Try lowering heels to floor without losing arch in low back. Relax stomach and hold for allotted time.

Downward Dog (Elevated)

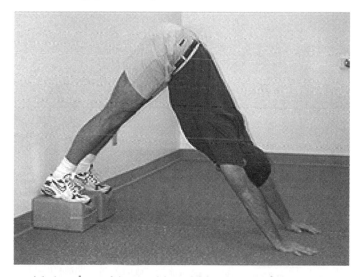

Start with hands and knees hip width apart and perpendicular to the floor. Curling toes under on 6" block, lift knees off floor by tightening quads and maintaining arch in low back. Without moving hands or feet, push head and chest through arms towards knees while still maintaining arch in low back and quad tight. Try lowering heels to floor without losing arch in low back. Relax stomach and hold for allotted time.

Elbow Press (Sitting)

Sitting in chair with knees bent at 90 degrees and hip width apart, roll hips forward pushing stomach out to create arch in low back. Place knuckles on temples with elbows pointing straight ahead. With elbows shoulder width apart, place strap just above elbows. Keeping shoulder blades squeezed together, press and release against strap. Keep stomach relaxed.

Elbow Press (Static Floor)

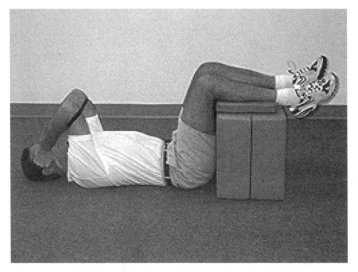

With legs propped on block and knees bent at 90 degrees, place knuckles on temples and elbows pointing towards ceiling. With elbows shoulder width apart, place strap just above elbows. Keeping shoulder blades squeezed together, press and release against strap. Keep stomach relaxed.

Elbow Rotations (Extended Floor Position)

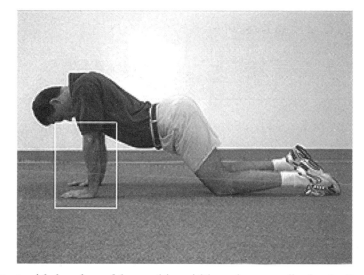

Start with hands and knees hip width and perpendicular to floor. Walk hands forward 4-6" and allow shoulders to reposition over hands without moving knees on floor. With hips now in front of knees, allow back to sway, shoulder blades to collapse together, and head to drop. While holding this position, keep arms straight and rotate elbows in and out keeping hands pointing straight ahead. RELAX STOMACH.

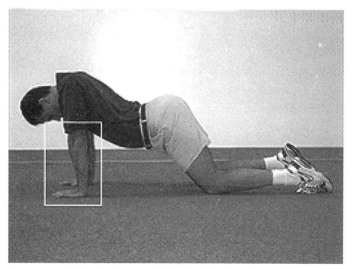

Elbow Rotations (Wall)

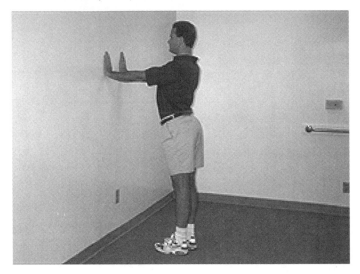

Facing wall, stand arms-length away and place palms on wall with fingers pointing straight up wall. Keeping arms straight allow shoulder blades to squeeze together and rotate elbows in and out. Make sure feet are hip width apart and straight ahead. Relax stomach and do not shrug shoulders.

Elevated Blocked Floor

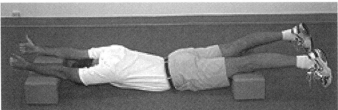

Lying on stomach, elevate arms and legs by placing 6" blocks under forearms and 3" above knees. keeping arms and legs extended hip width apart, point thumbs towards Elbow. **Elbow Press (Sitting)** Sitting in chair with knees bent at 90 degrees and hip width apart, roll hips forward pushing stomach out to create arch in low back. Place knuckles on temples with elbows pointing straight ahead. With elbows shoulder width apart, place strap just above elbows. Keeping shoulder blades squeezed together, press and release against strap. Keep stomach relaxed.

Elevated Cats and Dogs

Place knees on 14" block, hip width apart. Start with hands and knees hip width and perpendicular to floor. Walk hands forward 4-6" and allow shoulders to reposition over hands without moving knees on floor. Pull chin to chest while pushing low back to ceiling . Then look up to ceiling and allow back to sway and shoulder blades to pull back and together. Keep a constant, smooth motion not allowing your body to move forward or backwards.

Elevated Femur Rotations (Floor)

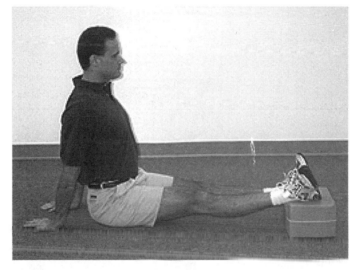

Sitting on floor with hands propped behind back, spread legs slightly wider than hip width and place one heel on 6" block. Keeping quads tight, toes pulled back and low back arched, rotate leg from hip in full range of motion without bending knee. Keep stomach and opposite leg relaxed. Switch legs after recommended amount of repetitions. Don't shrug shoulders.

Elevated Femur Rotations (Wall)

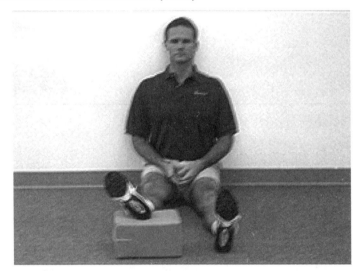

Sitting on floor with hips and back against wall, spread legs slightly wider than hip width and place one heel on 6" block. Keeping quads tight, toes pulled back and low back arched, rotate leg from hip in full range of motion without bending knee. Keep stomach and opposite leg relaxed. Switch legs after recommended amount of repetitions. Don't shrug shoulders and make sure not to pull elbows back, but keep shoulder blades squeezed together.

Extended Ankle Abduction

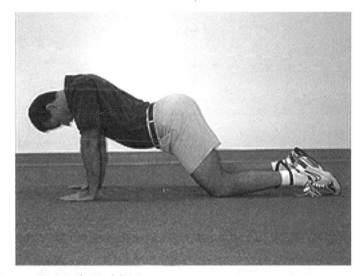

Start with hands and knees hip width and perpendicular to floor. Walk hands forward 4-6" and allow shoulders to reposition over hands without moving knees on floor. With hips now in front of knees, allow back to sway, shoulder blades to collapse together, and head to drop. While holding this position, press out on strap hip width at ankles and release. Feel contraction on the outside of hips. Breathe and relax stomach.

Extended Ankle Adduction

Start with hands and knees hip width and perpendicular to floor. Walk hands forward 4-6" and allow shoulders to reposition over hands without moving knees on floor. With hips now in front of knees, allow back to sway, shoulder blades to collapse together, and head to drop. While holding this position, squeeze and release pillow between ankles with both inside of heels and toes. Feel in glutes and back of legs.

Extended Floor

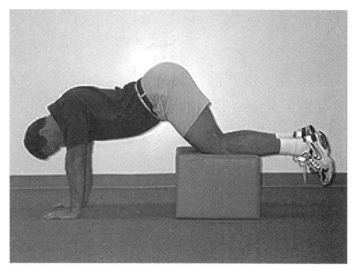

Place knees on 14" block, hip width apart. Start with hands and knees hip width and perpendicular to floor. Walk hands forward 4-6" and allow shoulders to reposition over hands without moving knees on floor. Let back sway with shoulder blades together and arms straight. Hold this position by pulling knees into block, keeping body from moving forward. Relax back of legs and stomach and allow head to drop.

Extended Floor Position

Start with hands and knees hip width and perpendicular to floor. Walk hands forward 4-6" and allow shoulders to reposition over hands without moving knees on floor. With hips now in front of knees, allow back to sway, shoulder blades to collapse together, and head to drop. Hold this position by pulling knees into floor, keeping body from moving forward. Relax back of legs and stomach and allow head to drop.

Extended Floor Position (Elbows)

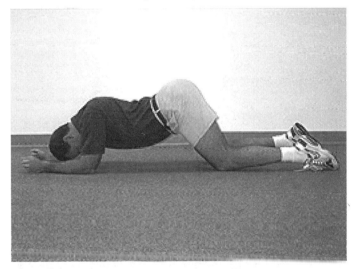

Start with hands and knees hip width and perpendicular to floor. Walk hands forward 4-6" and allow shoulders to reposition over hands without moving knees on floor. Once in this position, re-place elbows where your hands are. With hips now in front of knees, allow back to sway, shoulder blades to collapse together, and head to drop. Hold this position by pulling knees into floor, keeping body from moving forward. Relax back of legs and stomach..

Extended Floor Position (Active)

Start with hands and knees hip width and perpendicular to floor. Walk hands forward 4-6" and allow shoulders to reposition over hands without moving knees on floor. With hips now in front of knees, allow back to sway, shoulder blades to collapse together, and head to drop. While in this position pull knees into floor, spread forearms apart and push butt backwards keeping sway in back. Feel stretch in shoulders and down the mid back. Relax back of legs and stomach.

Extended Supine

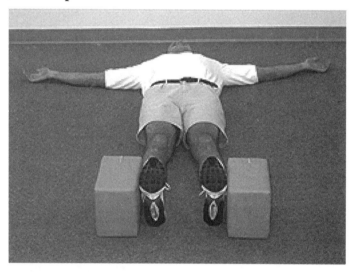

Lie on back with arms straight out to sides, palms up. Keep knees and feet hip width apart and pointed towards the ceiling the whole time. Relaxing the upper body, abdominals and quadriceps, actively pull back toes for the allotted amount of time. IMPORTANT: keep feet straight up and DO NOT let them splay out to the side. If needed, place 2 pillows on the outside of the feet o keep them properly aligned. Do not let feet lean against pillows.

Extended Supine (Ankle/Knee Press)

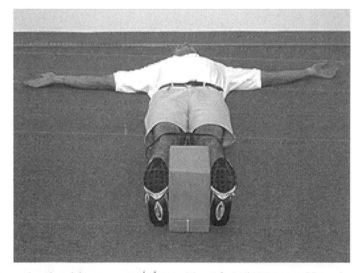

Lie on back with arms straight out to sides, palms up. Keep knees and feet hip width apart and pointed towards the ceiling the whole time. Relaxing the upper body, abdominals and quadriceps, actively pull back toes for the allotted amount of time. While holding this position actively hold out against strap at knees (6" apart) and hold in on block at feet. Relax stomach and upper body, feel in hips and let back relax into floor.

Extended Supine (Ankle/Knee Opposite)

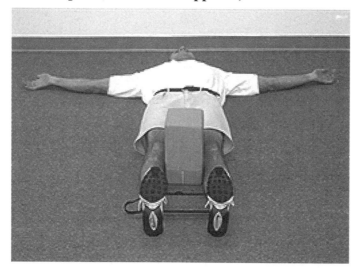

Lie on back with arms straight out to sides, palms up. keep knees and feet hip width apart and pointed towards the ceiling the whole time. Relaxing the upper body, abdominals and quadriceps, actively pull back toes for the allotted amount of time. While holding this position actively hold out against strap at ankles (6" apart) and hold in on block at knees. Relax stomach and upper body, feel in hips and let back relax into floor.

Extended Triangle

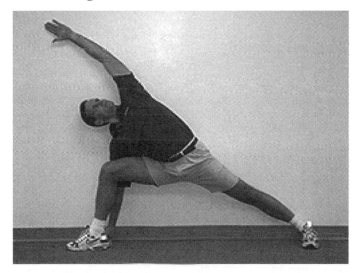

Standing against wall, place left foot perpendicular to wall with heel touching wall. Placing right foot parallel to wall (about 3"away), take a large step to the right. Keeping left quad tight and both glutes against wall, slowly bend until right knee is directly over ankle 3" off wall. Keeping both shoulders on wall with arms straight and palms facing out, slowly bend torso from waist towards right knee. Place right hand between right ankle and wall while slowly taking left arm overhead towards the right. Hold position for allotted amount of time and breathe!

Flamingo Stretch

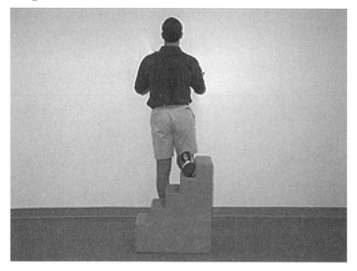

Stand with feet straight and hip width, hands resting on wall or back of chair. Place one foot on back of chair keeping upper body relaxed the whole time. Weight should be evenly distributed between legs. Curl hips under to feel stretch in thigh on bent leg. Don't let hip shift out to side on the straight leg keeping hips level.

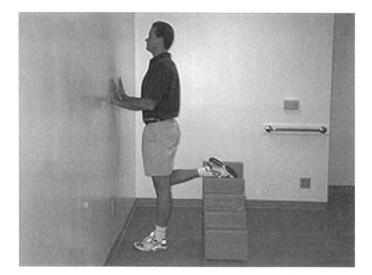

Floor Clock

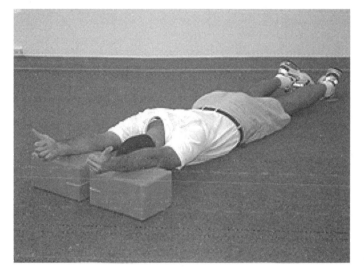

In prone position with legs straight and feet pigeon toed, place forearms on 6" blocks with arms overhead. Keeping arms straight with light fists, externally rotate shoulders pointing thumbs towards ceiling. With forehead resting on floor, relax stomach and glutes allowing heels to fall out to side. Hold for allotted time then move blocks out to side so that arms are at a 45 degree angle from shoulders. Again hold position for allotted time then move blocks to place arms at a 90 degree angle from side and hold. Emphasize rotation from shoulders and keep rest of body relaxed.

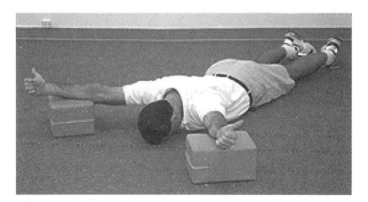

Floor Presses (Hooklying)

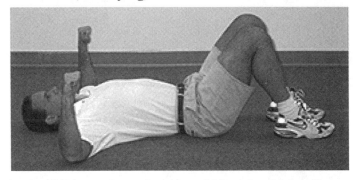

On back with knees bent, feet hip width and straight, place arms straight out to side and bend elbows to 90 degrees pointing fists to ceiling. Without rotating from shoulders, press elbows into floor and feel shoulder blades squeeze together, then release. Relax stomach and breathe.

Floor Presses (Inverted Wall)

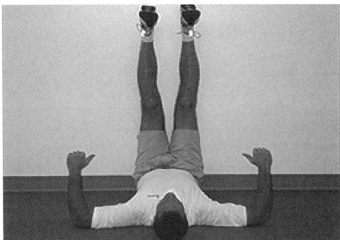

Lie on back with legs straight up on wall, feet hip width apart. With quads tight, position body away from wall, if necessary, so that tail bone rests on floor. Keep knees pointed away from wall and toes flexed back. Place arms straight out to side and bend elbows to 90 degrees pointing fists to ceiling. Without rotating from shoulders, press elbows into floor and feel shoulder blades squeeze together, then release. Relax stomach and breathe.

Floor Presses (Lying Groin Stretch)

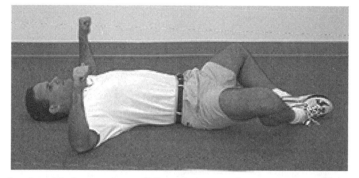

On back with knees bent, place feet together and allow knees to separate apart until bottom of soles come together. Place arms straight out to side and bend elbows to 90 degrees pointing fists to ceiling. Without rotating from shoulders, press elbows into floor and feel shoulder blades squeeze together, then release. Relax stomach and breathe.

Floor Presses (Static Floor)

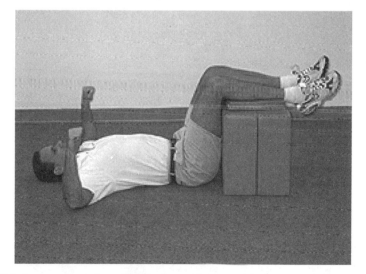

With legs propped on block, knees bent at 90 degrees, place arms straight out to side and bend elbows to 90 degrees pointing fists to ceiling. Without rotating from shoulders, press elbows into floor and feel shoulder blades squeeze together, then release. Relax stomach and breathe.

Free Crunches

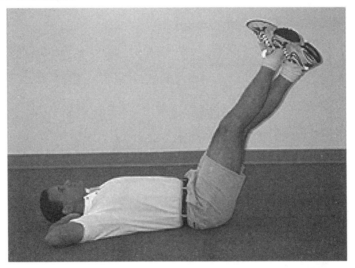

On back, cross ankles and lift legs to 70 degree position from floor keeping leg slightly bent. With hands interlaced behind head, look backwards and lift elbows, shoulders and head off floor using abdominal muscles. Then return to starting position with elbows, shoulders and head touching floor. Switch ankle position when indicated.

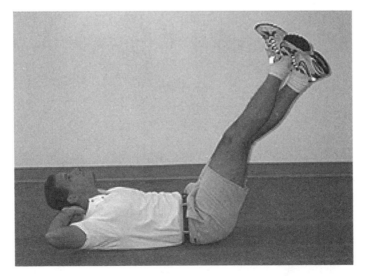

Free Fall

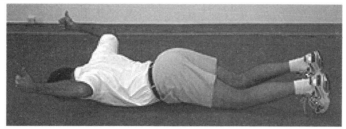

Lying on stomach with forehead resting on floor, pull toes under and place arms out to side with elbows bent at 90 degrees, thumbs pointing to ceiling. Digging knees into floor, allow back to arch pushing buttocks to ceiling and lift arms up to ceiling maintaining 90 degrees. Lift arms by pulling shoulder blades together and keep fists as high off floor as possible. Relax head and stomach and hold for allotted time.

Full Back Bend

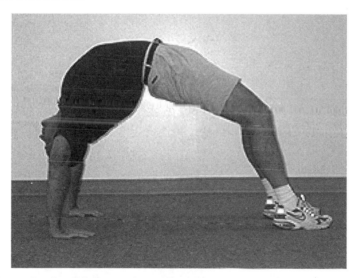

Lie on back with knees bent, feet hip width and straight. Place hands above head with palms flat on floor, fingers pointing to-wards feet. Lift hips off floor extending arms as much as possible while keeping knees hip width. Push hips as far off floor as pos-sible and hold position for allotted time.

Full Sit-ups

On back with knees bent, feet hip width and straight, interlace hands behind head keeping elbows back on floor. With feet secured, keep back arched and pull torso off floor using hip flexors. Keep head looking back to maintain extension and roll hips forward at top of sit up. Maintain arch in back, elbows pulled back and lower torso to floor trying to touch shoulders first. Then repeat.

Full Squat

Hold on to waist-high support, (sink, open door, etc.), with feet hip width and straight and close to support base. Allowing arms to straighten, arch back and sit down holding back into extension and keeping knees directly over ankles. Hold for allotted time.

Glute Squeezes

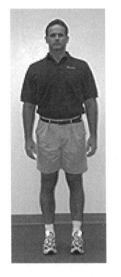 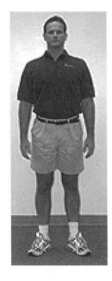

Standing with feet hip width and straight, squeeze buttocks together and release without tightening stomach or thighs. If you find it difficult to isolate your glute muscles, then stand with your feet pointed out for the first set.

Groin Stretch

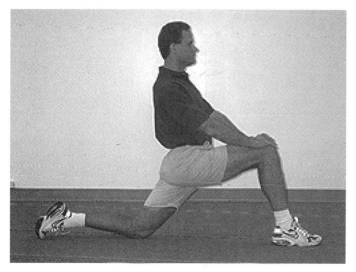

In kneeling position, place one foot in front of the other keeping feet hip width apart. Place interlaced hands on front knee or on head as instructed, to keep torso in upright position. Lunge forward not letting knee extend in front of ankle. Feel in groin.

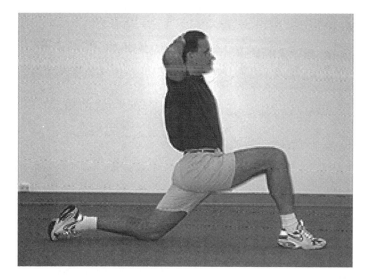

Gravity Drop

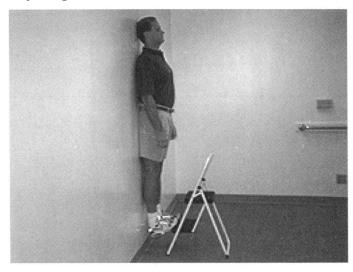

Standing on an incline board or step ladder against wall with legs straight, keep feet straight and hip width. Relax stomach and let body weight sink into heels. Feel a stretch in calves. Breathe!

Gravity Drop (Wall)

Placing balls of feet on edge of stair step or edge of step ladder, hold onto railing at side or door jam in front. Allowing arms to be straight, let body feel like it is leaning back with stomach relaxed and arch in back. Keep body (joints) vertical, legs straight, and allow heels to drop towards floor. Hold position for allotted time. Don't shrug shoulders.

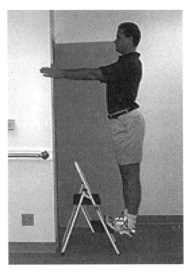

Hamstring Curls

Stand on both feet with hands resting on wall or back of chair.
Point toe into ground and curl leg from knee towards buttocks.
Return leg to floor, touch toe to floor, and repeat. Do not let knee
move forward when curling leg and keep hips squared at all times.
relax shoulders and stomach.

Handle Stretch

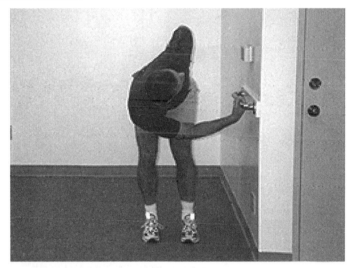

Stand sideways to door handle with feet hip width and straight.
Slightly bend at knees, arch low back and grab handle underneath
with hand furthest away from door. Place back of hand of other
arm on small of back. Keeping hips square, knees bent, rotate
torso by opening up the inside shoulder towards the ceiling, NOT
allowing the hips to move. Keep knees hip width and parallel
throughout exercise. Hold for allotted time then switch.

Handstand

Stand on hands with knees facing the wall. Push arms into floor until elbows lock. Hands should be no more than 6" away from wall keeping stomach off wall. Keep quads fairly tight and hold position.

Heel-Toe (Block)

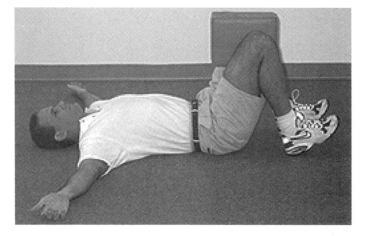

On back with knees bent, feet hip width and straight, place pillow between knees, press in and hold. Simultaneously, lift just heels off floor then just toes in a rocking motion and repeat for allotted reps. Relax stomach and breathe.

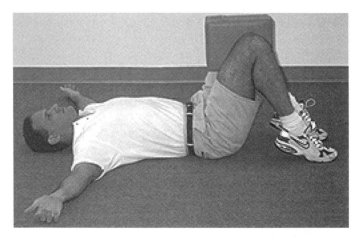

Heel/Toe (Strap)

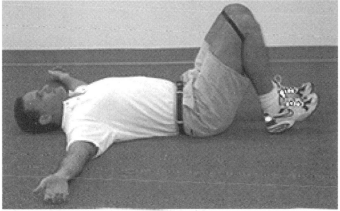

On back with knees bent, feet hip width and straight, place strap around knees, press out and hold. Simultaneously, lift just heels off floor then just toes in a rocking motion and repeat for allotted reps. Relax stomach and breathe.

Hip Abduction

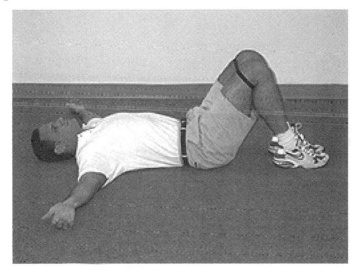

On back with knees bent, place strap around knees either together or hip width. With feet straight press out against strap and release, relaxing stomach and shoulders. Breathe!

Hip Abduction (Standing)

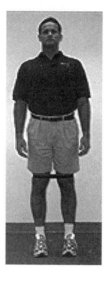

Standing with feet close together, place strap around knees. Then position feet hip width to make strap snug. While keeping legs from bending and stomach relaxed, press out and release against strap using outside of hips and not by rolling out on feet. Relax shoulders and breathe.

Hip Abduction (Static)

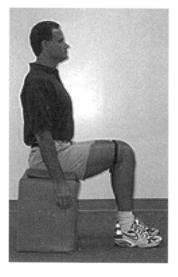

Hip Abduction (Static Floor)—With legs propped on block, knees bent at 90 degrees, place strap around knees either hip width or together. While relaxing stomach and shoulders press and release against strap.

Hip Abduction/Adduction

On back with knees and hips bent at 90 degrees, place feet hip width and straight on wall. KEEPING FEET STRAIGHT slowly spread knees apart while pivoting on outside of feet keeping heels on wall, then bring knees together. Relax stomach.

Hip Adduction (Hooklying)

On back with knees bent, feet flat on floor. Place 6" block between knees, press and release, feeling in inner thighs. Relax stomach.

Hip Adduction (Gravity Drop)

Standing on an incline board or step ladder against wall with legs straight, keep feet straight and hip width. Relax stomach and let body weight sink into heels. Feel a stretch in calves. Breathe! Place 6" block between knees, press and release, feeling in inner thighs. Relax stomach.

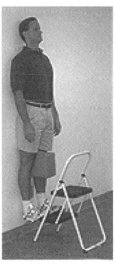

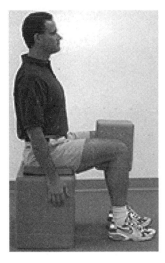

Hip Adduction (Sitting)

Sitting half way off chair, create arch in low back by rolling hips forward and pushing stomach out. Keep knees and feet hip-width apart with feet pointed straight ahead. Place 6" block between knees, press and release, feeling in inner thighs. Relax stomach.

Hip Adduction (Standing)

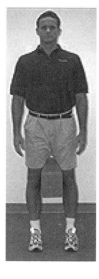

Stand erect with knees and feet hip width apart, feet pointing straight ahead. Place 6" block between knees, press and release, feeling in inner thighs. Relax stomach.

Hip Adduction (Static Floor)

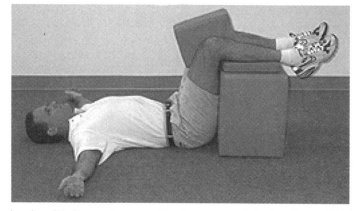

On back with knees bent at 90 degrees on block, place 6" block between knees, press and release, feeling in inner thighs. Relax stomach.

Hip Thrusts

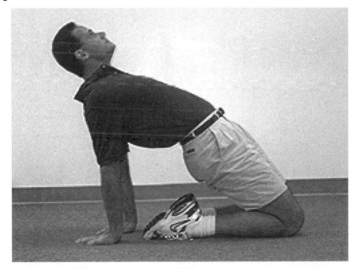

Kneel on floor with knees and ankles hip width. Place hands behind on floor and sit back on heels. Thrust hips up to ceiling arching back, pushing stomach out. Then return back to sitting on heels. Repeat for allotted reps.

Hurdle Stretch

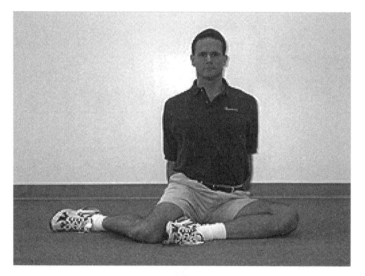

Sitting on floor with hips square, bend one knee in front on floor with foot in, bend the other knee 90 degrees placing foot out to side. Prop hands behind for minor support and roll hips forward as much as possible while trying to maintain even pressure on buttocks on floor. Hold for allotted time. Then switch leg position.

Intercostal Stretch

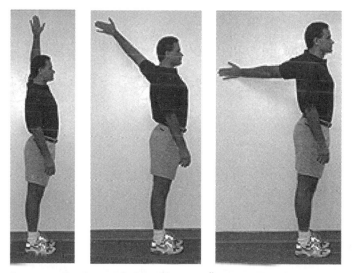

Stand perpendicular with feet 1' away from wall. Place arm closest to wall straight up with palm on wall and hold for allotted time
without twisting body. Repeat sequence at 45 and 90 degrees.
Maintain feet and hips straight entire time. When completed with
all positions, switch to other side. BREATHE.

Inverted Rotations

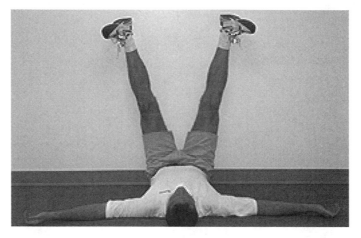

Lie on back with hips and back of legs against wall. Separate feet until they are just wider than shoulder width apart. Keeping thighs tight with toes pulled back, rotate entire leg from hip in and out. Move away from wall if buttocks lifts off floor. After allotted reps, spread legs apart about 1' wider and repeat. Then spread legs as wide as possible and perform last set. Keep upper body and stomach relaxed.

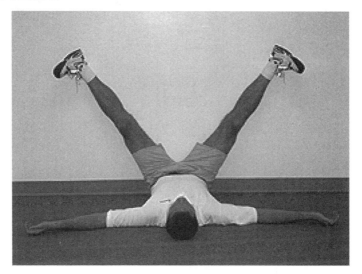

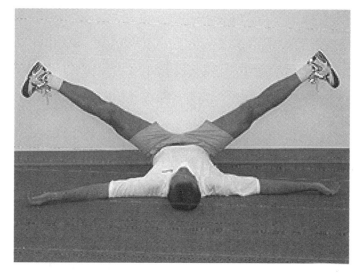

Inverted Splits

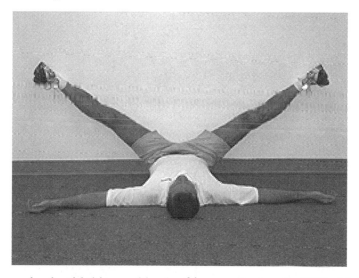

Lie on back with hips and back of legs against wall. With thighs tight and toes pulled back, separate feet and legs as wide as possible. Rotate knees inward trying to point them at each other. Keep upper body and stomach relaxed. Breathe.

Inverted Wall

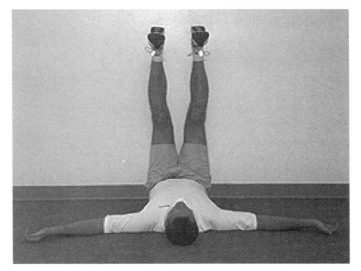

Lie on back with legs straight up on wall, feet hip width apart. With quads tight, position body away from wall, if necessary, so that tail bone rests on floor. Keeping knees pointed away from wall and toes flexed back., feel stretch in hamstrings and relax stomach.

Joggers Stretch

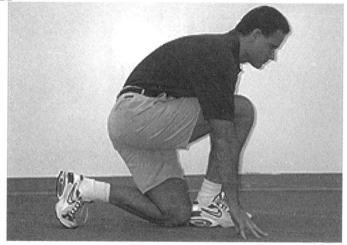

With right foot flat on floor, kneel down placing left knee directly behind right knee. Curl left toes under, making sure that feet are straight and directly in line with each other. Place hands on floor and stand up keeping quads tight and back flat, placing feet flat on floor without changing foot position. Keep hips square by not allowing them to rotate. Shoulders and stomach should remain relaxed. Hold for allotted amount of time and return to kneeling position when finished.

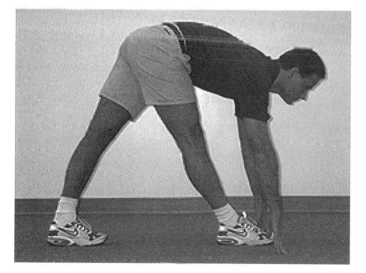

Joggers Stretch (Assisted)

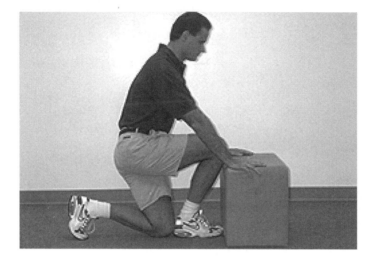

With right foot flat on floor, kneel down placing left knee directly behind right knee. Curl left toes under making sure that feet are straight and directly in line with each other. Place hands on chair and stand up keeping quads tight and back flat, placing feet flat on floor without changing foot position. Keep hips square by not allowing them to rotate. Shoulders and stomach should remain relaxed. Hold for allotted amount of time and return to kneeling position when finished.

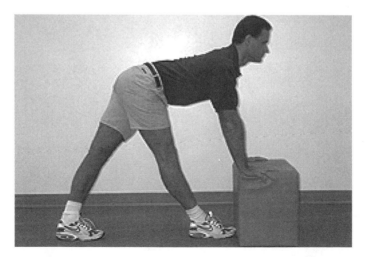

Knee Extensions

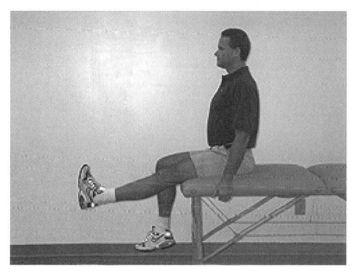

Sitting on table with feet off floor, create arch in low back by roll-ing hips forward and pushing stomach out. Fully try to extend knee by tightening quadricep without losing arch in low back. Feel in hamstring as knee is extended. Relax stomach and breathe.

Kneeling Ankle Press (Block)

On knees (hip width)with body in an upright position, place 6" block between ankles. Press and release inside of tocs and heels into block feeling contraction in back of leg and buttocks. Relax stomach.

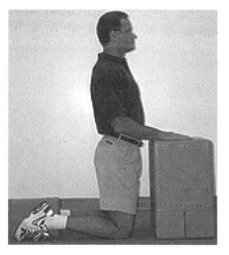

Kneeling Ankle Press (Strap)

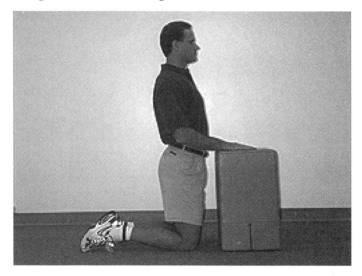

On knees (hip width) with body in an upright position, place strap around ankles. Press out and release against strap feeling contraction in the outside of hips. Relax stomach.

Kneeling Clock

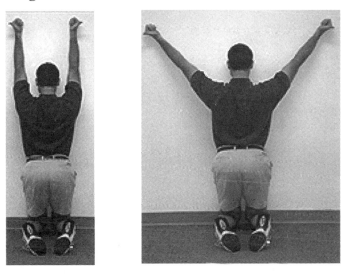

Kneeling on floor with knees hip width and touching wall, lay tops of feet flat and pigeon toed. Relax forehead against wall. Place arms straight overhead, make a slight fist with thumbs pointing at each other, and rotate entire arms from the shoulder so that the thumbs are pointing away from wall. Let hips move away from wall, stomach relaxed, to feel quads working, and arch in low back. Hold arms straight overhead, 45 and 90 degrees for 1 minute in each position.

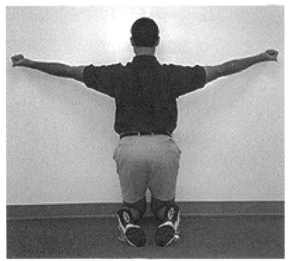

Kneeling Overhead Extension

Place knees hip width on floor with feet pigeon toed behind. Interlace fingers together, push palms away from body so that arms become straight and locked at elbows. While pulling shoulder blades together, slowly raise locked arms over head while keeping upper torso from leaning back. Allowing stomach to relax and fall out, feel arch in low back. Do not let arms bend or shoulders shrug, constantly pulling arms back with head relaxed back looking up at hands.

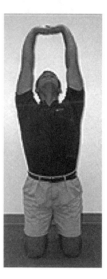

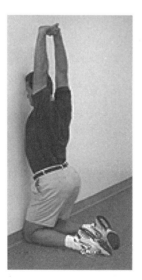

Kneeling Overhead Extension (Wall)

Kneeling on floor with knees hip width and touching wall, lay tops of feet flat and pigeon toed. Relax forehead against wall. Place arms straight overhead, interlace fingers together and push palms to ceiling locking arms and pulling arms off wall as far as possible. Let hips move away from wall, stomach relaxed, to feel quads working, and arch in low back. Do not shrug shoulders and make sure to breathe!

Kneeling Overhead Stretch

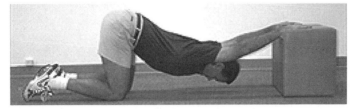

Kneeling on floor with knees and feet hip width, place forearms on 18" block. Keeping hips directly over knees, allow head, back and stomach to fall to the floor by letting back sway, and stomach relax. Keep arms straight and take deep breaths, sinking closer to floor after every exhalation.

Kneeling Overhead Stretch (Crossed)

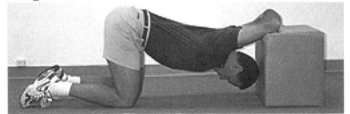

Kneeling on floor with knees and feet hip width, place forearms on 18" block. Bend elbows to 90 degrees and allow forearms to rest each other placing either hand on opposite elbow Keeping hips directly over knees, allow head, back and stomach to fall to the floor by letting back sway, and stomach relax. Take deep breaths, sinking closer to floor after every exhalation.

Kneeling Wall Press

Kneeling on floor with knees 6" from wall, place hands chest high and in push-up position on wall. Curl toes under feet so that bottom of toes are flat on floor. Pushing off toes, resist forward momentum by stabilizing hands against wall. Don't move any part of body while pressing toes into floor. Feel contraction in low back and quads. Relax stomach.

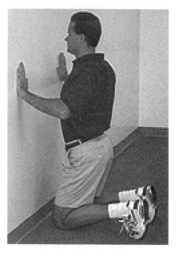

Lower Spinal Floor Twist

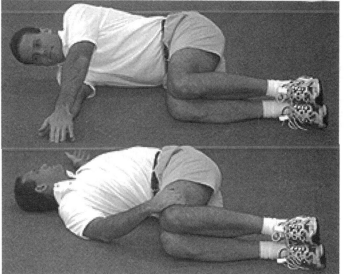

Lying on floor in fetal position, keep knees and arms at 90 degrees, hands together. KEEPING KNEES FROM SLIDING APART, open arms allowing top arm to relax toward the floor on the other side (open like a book) head turns with arm. Relax stomach. Concentrate on breathing and feel upper torso sink to floor on every exhalation without knees sliding apart. Remain in exercise until shoulder reaches the floor or your body stops sinking to floor.

Lying Calf/Hamstring Stretch

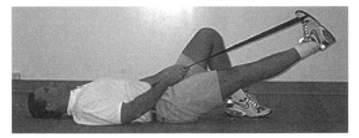

Lying on back with one leg bent and the other straight out, place strap around the ball of foot of the extended leg. Tighten leg , raise whole leg off floor about 1' and pull back on strap promoting a stretch in calf muscle. Do not bend knee. After 1 minute move strap down to arch of foot and slowly raise leg up to ceiling as far as you can WITHOUT bending knee to promote stretch in hamstring. Hold for 1 minute. In each position make sure to relax shoulders and stomach and concentrate on breathing.

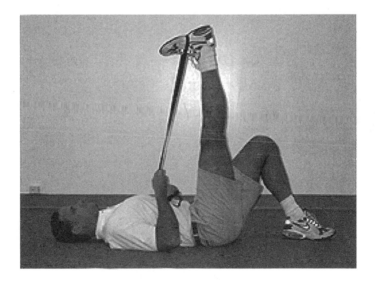

Lying Floor Twist

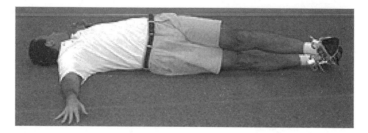

On back with legs extended (hip width), place left heel on right big toe. Keeping quads tight and toes pulled back, allow feet to rotate to the right by lifting left hip to ceiling. Place arms to side, palms down, keep stomach and shoulders relaxed while looking the opposite direction. Hold position for allotted time and switch direction, rotating to the other side.

Lying Groin Stretch

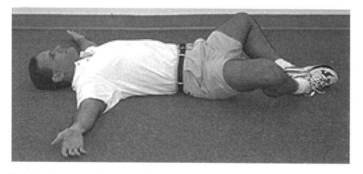

On back with knees bent, place feet together and allow knees to apart until bottom of soles come together. Feel back slightly arch while allowing legs to stretch to floor. Keep arms out to side and relax whole body. Breathe.

Lying Hip Flexor Stretch

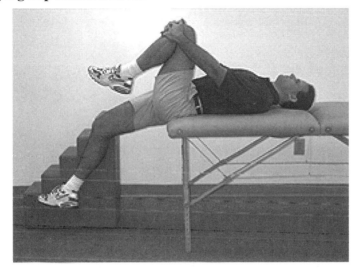

Lying on back with tailbone on edge of table, interlace hands behind knee and pull towards same-side shoulder allowing other leg to drop to floor. Prop leg at side to keep from falling outward. Feel stretch in front of hip, relax shoulders and breathe.

Lying Leg Rotations

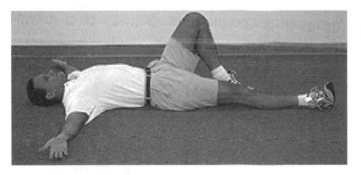

Lie on back with one leg bent and the other straight and aligned on floor. Keeping thigh tight with toes pulled back, rotate entire leg in and out from hip. Keep stomach relaxed and upper body relaxed. Place bent leg on 18" block or chair if instructed by therapist.

Oblique Crunches

On back with knees and hips at 90 degrees, place feet straight and hip width on wall. While looking back, raise elbows, shoulders and head together off floor. Then twist towards opposite knee while keeping elbows pulled back the whole time. Return to starting position and repeat.

Overhead Extension (Buddha's Pose)

Sitting back on heels with knees together, induce arch in low back by rolling hips forward and not by leaning back. Interlace fingers together, push palms away from body so that arms become straight and locked at elbows. While pulling shoulder blades together, slowly raise locked arms over head while keeping upper torso from leaning back. Allowing stomach to relax and fall out, feel arch in low back. Do not let arms bend OR shoulders shrug, constantly pulling arms back with head relaxed back looking up at hands.

Overhead Extension (Sitting)

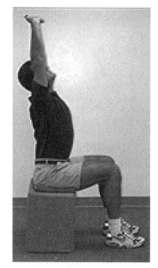

Sitting on chair with knees bent at 90 degrees, feet straight, induce arch in low back by rolling hips forward and not by leaning back. Interlace fingers together. Push palms away from body so that arms become straight and locked at elbows. While pulling shoulder blades together. Slowly raise locked arms over head while keeping upper torso from leaning back. Allowing stomach to relax and fall out, feel arch in low back. Do not let arms bend OR shoulders shrug, constantly pulling arms back with head relaxed back looking up at hands.

Overhead Extension (Standing)

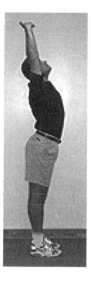

Stand with feet straight and hip width. Interlace fingers together, push palms away from body so that arms become straight and locked at elbows. While pulling shoulder blades together, slowly raise locked arms over head while keeping upper torso from leaning back. Allowing stomach to relax and fall out, feel arch in low back. Do not let arms bend OR shoulders shrug, constantly pulling arms back with head relaxed back looking up at hands. Keep thighs tight placing weight on the balls of feet.

Overhead Press (Hooklying)

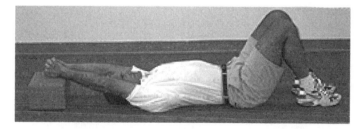

On back with knees bent, feet hip width and straight, clasp hands together with arms straight and place them on 6" block behind head. Press and release hands into block without bending elbows. Feel shoulder blades squeeze together . Relax stomach and breathe.

Overhead Press (Inverted Wall)

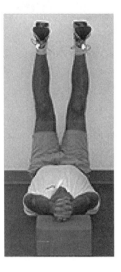

Lie on back with legs straight up on wall, feet hip width apart. With quads tight, position body away from wall, if necessary, so that tail bone rests on floor. Keeping knees pointed away from wall and toes flexed back, clasp hands together with arms straight and place them on 6" block behind head. Press and release hands into block without bending elbows. Feel shoulder blades squeeze together. Relax stomach and breathe.

Overhead Press (Lying Groin Stretch)

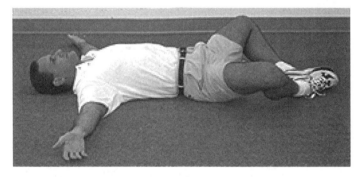

On back with knees bent, place feet together and allow knees to apart until bottom of soles come together. Feel back slightly arch while allowing legs to stretch to floor. Keep arms out to side and relax whole body. Clasp hands together with arms straight and place them on 6" block behind head. Press and release hands into block without bending elbows. Feel shoulder blades squeeze together . Relax stomach and breathe.

Overhead Press (Static Floor)

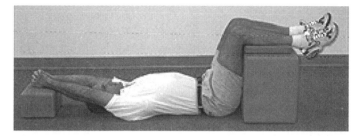

On back with knees bent at 90 degrees on 18" block, clasp hands together with arms straight and place them on 6" block behind head. Press and release hands into block without bending elbows. Feel shoulder blades squeeze together . Relax stomach and breathe.

Outer Thigh Lift

Lying on side with head propped in hand, elbow on floor, extend body as straight as possible. Bend leg closest to floor to 90 degrees, tighten other leg and pull toes back. Rotate straightened leg by pointing knee to floor then raise leg to ceiling and back down again without rotating hips. Keep upper body relaxed.

Pec Stretch

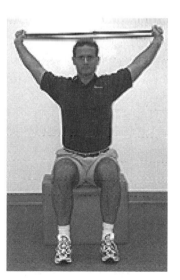

Sitting with knees bent at 90 degrees, feet and knees straight and hip width, hold onto strap wider than shoulder width. Keeping arms straight, elbows locked, slowly raise arms over head and behind head without leaning torso backwards or forwards. Maintain arch in low back and keep stomach relaxed. Return arms back to staring position in same manner and repeat.

Pelvic Bridge (Or Active)

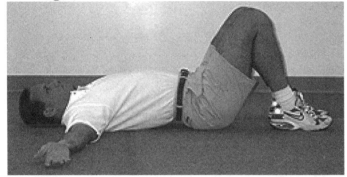

Lie on back with knees bent (hip width) and feet flat on floor. Relax arms at side. Keeping feet flat on floor lift pelvis towards ceiling using buttocks, hamstrings, and lower back. If exercise calls for active bridges, then raise and lower pelvis for allotted amount of times.

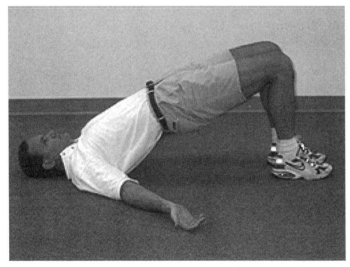

Pelvic Tilts

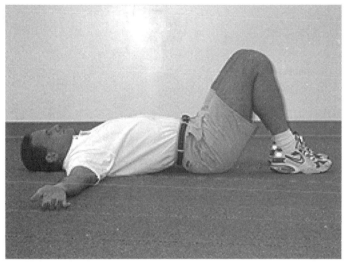

Lie on back with knees bent (hip width) and feet flat on floor. Relax arms at side. Flatten low back into floor by rolling hips backwards. Then, roll hips in opposite direction to create arch in low back. Keep legs relaxed during entire exercise. Motion of pelvic tilts are continuous.

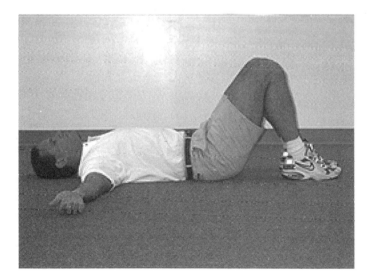

Piriformis Stretch

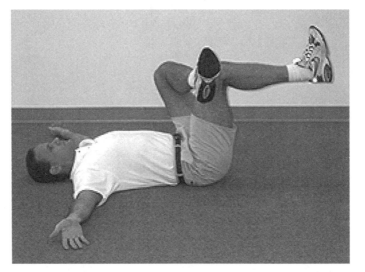

Lie on back with knees bent, feet on floor, hip width. Cross right ankle to left knee and lift left foot off floor bending knee to 90 degrees. Press right knee away and pull left toes back. Keep back from rotating to one side or the other and breathe, relaxing stomach as much as possible.

Piriformis Stretch (Crossover)

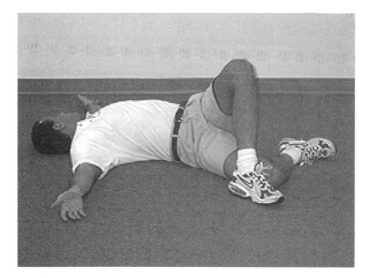

Lie on back with knees bent, feet on floor, hip width. Cross right ankle to left knee. Pivot off outside of left foot and rotate right foot and left knee to floor as one unit. keeping right foot flat on floor, press right knee slightly away feeling stretch on outside of right hip. Place arms out to side, relax shoulders and stomach and look the opposite direction.

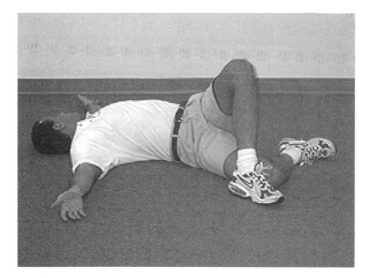

Piriformis Stretch (Floor)

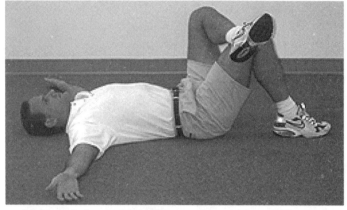

Lie on back with knees bent, feet on floor , hip width. Cross right ankle to left knee. Keeping hips square, press right knee away relaxing stomach and shoulders. Feel in right glute.

Piriformis Stretch (Heel/Toe)

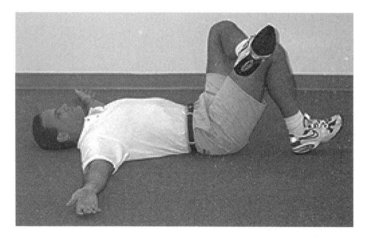

Lie on back with knees bent, feet on floor, hip width. Cross right ankle to left knee. Keeping hips square, press right knee away relaxing stomach and shoulders. Feel in right glute. While maintaining this position take foot on floor and lift toes up keeping heel on floor, then lift heel up keeping toes on floor. Repeat for allotted amount of times.

Piriformis Stretch (Wall)

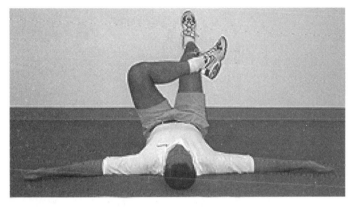

Lie on back with knees bent at 90 degrees, feet hip width on wall. Cross right ankle to left knee. Keeping hips square, press right knee away relaxing stomach and shoulders. Feel in right glute.

Prone Ankle Press (Block-MFB)

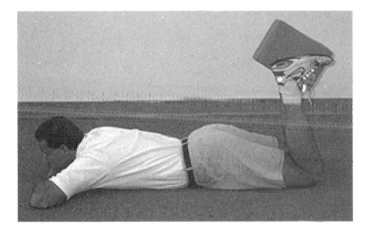

Lie on stomach with arms propped up on 6" blocks. Place arms straight out from sides with elbows bent at 90 degrees. With feet pigeon toed, let buttocks and low back relax allowing hips to settle into floor. Breathe. With knees bent at 90 degrees. Place 6" block between feet. Evenly press and release into block with the inside border of each foot. Feel in buttocks. Relax stomach.

Prone Ankle Press (Strap)

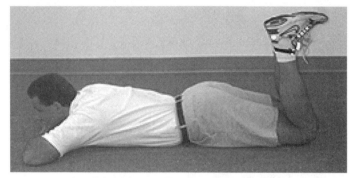

Lie on stomach with chin resting on hands, knees bent at 90 degrees. Place strap around ankles with knees and feet hip width apart. Evenly press and release ankles against strap. Feel in outer hip. Relax stomach.

Prone Ankle Press (Strap-MFB)

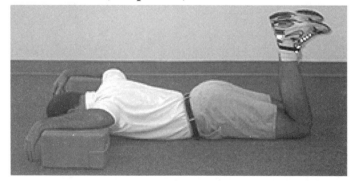

Lie on stomach with arms propped up on 6" blocks. Place arms straight out from sides with elbows bent at 90 degrees. With feet pigeon toed, let buttocks and low back relax allowing hips to settle into floor. Breathe. With knees bent at 90 degrees. Place strap around ankles with knees and feet hip width apart. Evenly press and release ankles against strap. Feel in outer hip. Relax stomach.

Prone Blocked Floor

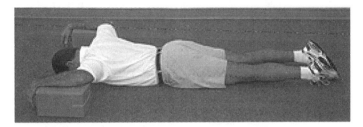

Lie on stomach with arms propped up on 6" blocks. Place arms straight out from sides with elbows bent at 90 degrees. With feet pigeon toed, let buttocks and low back relax allowing hips to settle into floor. Breathe.

Prone Knee Press

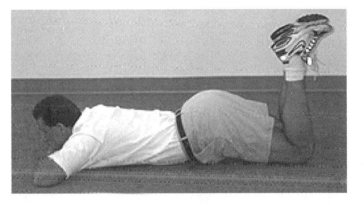

Lie on stomach with chin resting on hands. Bend knees to 90 de-grees keeping them hip width, and evenly press knees into floor using front of hips. Feel low back arch and hips lift off floor as knees press into floor. Relax stomach.

Prone Knee Press (MFB)

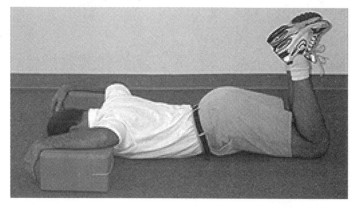

Lie on stomach with arms propped up on 6" blocks. Place arms straight out from sides with elbows bent at 90 degrees. With feet pigeon toed, let buttocks and low back relax allowing hips to settle into floor. Breathe. Bend knees to 90 degrees keeping them hip width, and evenly press knees into floor using front of hips. Feel low back arch and hips lift off floor as knees press into floor. Relax stomach.

Prone Knee Press (Unilateral)

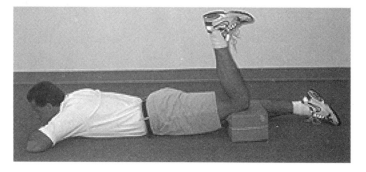

On stomach with chin resting on hands, bend one knee to 90 degrees and prop up on 6" block with the other leg straight out on floor. Press bent knee into block using front of hip. Keep other leg and stomach relaxed. Feel hips settle into floor evenly.

Prone Leg Curls (Block)

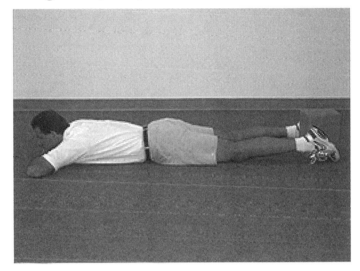

Lie on stomach with chin resting on hands, legs straight, feet on floor. Place 6" block between feet. Gently squeeze block while bending knees as much as possible and then lowering feet back to floor. Feel in hamstrings and glutes.

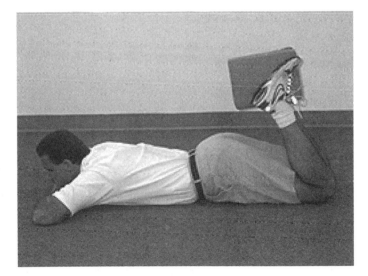

Prone Leg Curls (Block-MFB)

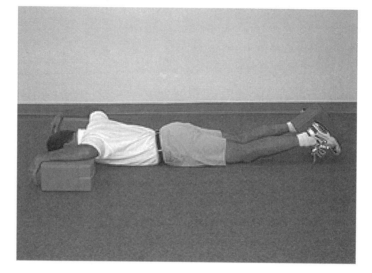

Lie on stomach with arms propped up on 6" blocks. Place arms straight out from sides with elbows bent at 90 degrees. With feet pigeon toed, let buttocks and low back relax allowing hips to settle into floor. Breathe. With legs straight, feet on floor, place 6" block between feet. Gently squeeze block while bending knees as much as possible and then lowering feet back to floor. feel in hamstrings and glutes.

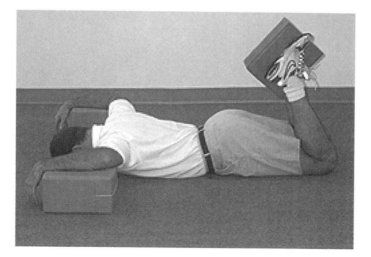

Prone Leg Curls (Strap)

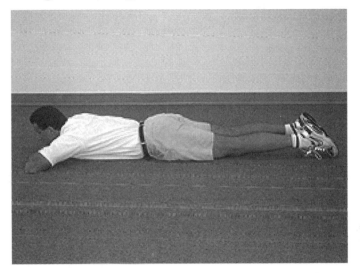

Lie on stomach with chin resting on hands, legs straight, feet on floor. Place strap around ankles with knees and feet hip width apart. Gently press out against strap and bend knees as much as possible, then lower feet back to floor. Feel in hamstrings and outer hips. Relax stomach.

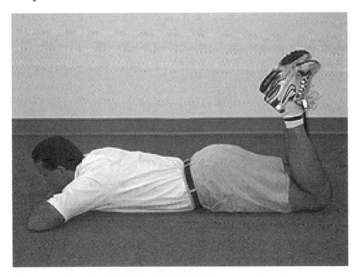

Prone Leg Curls (Strap-MFB)

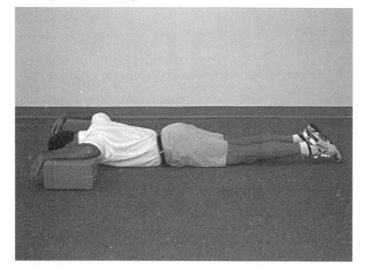

Lie on stomach with arms propped up on 6" blocks. Place arms straight out from sides with elbows bent at 90 degrees. With feet pigeon toed, let buttocks and low back relax allowing hips to settle into floor. Breathe. Place strap around ankles with knees and feet hip width apart. Gently press out against strap and bend knees as much as possible. Then lower feet back to floor. Feel in hamstrings and outer hips. Relax stomach.

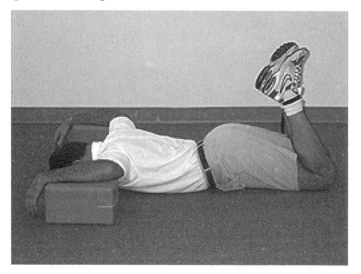

Prone Leg Raise

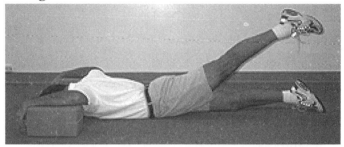

In Prone Blocked Position straighten one leg and slowly raise leg off ground while relaxing other leg. Hold leg off floor for 10 seconds while relaxing whole upper body. Alternate legs for allotted reps. Relax stomach and breathe.

Prone Opposite Blocked

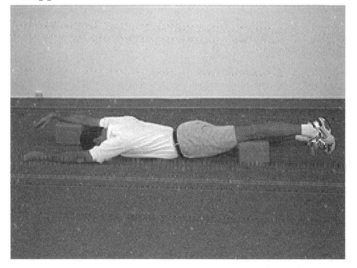

Lying on stomach with legs straight back and arms straight overhead, place 6" lift under forearm and 6" lift under opposite thigh just above knee. Rest forehead on floor and allow whole body to relax. Concentrate on breathing and let elevated hip settle into floor on every exhalation. Hold until hip stops sinking or is settled on floor.

Prone Opposite Glides

Lying on stomach with legs straight back and arms straight ahead, reach one arm forward while extending the opposite leg back. keep hips from rotating and hold position for allotted time, then switch.

Prone Opposite Lifts

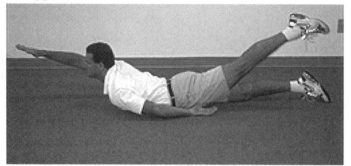

Lie on stomach with one arm straight ahead and the other at side with palm to ceiling. Lift the extended arm and the opposite leg straight up as high as possible while relaxing the other arm and leg. Look up at extended arm and hold for allotted time, then switch.

Prone Opposite Lifts (Hands and Knees)

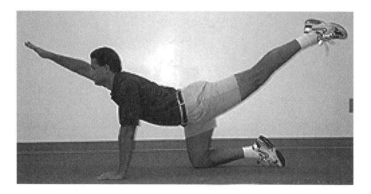

On hands and knees with knees directly under hips and hands under shoulders. Lift right arm and the opposite leg straight up as high as possible while relaxing the other arm and leg. Look up at extended arm and hold for allotted time, then switch.

Prone Scissors

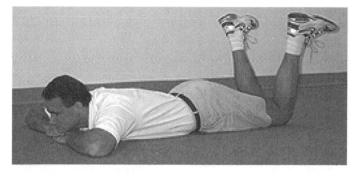

Lie on stomach and rest chin on hands. Knees bent and together, slowly let feet fall apart from each other, then bring feet together again. Relax stomach.

Prone Scissors (PBF)

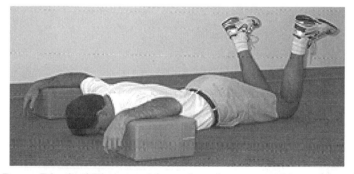

In Prone Blocked Floor position, place knees together and bend at 90 degrees. Slowly let feet fall apart from each other, and hold feeling arch in low back. Relax stomach.

Psoas Stretch

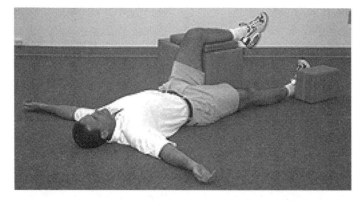

Lying on back with one leg up on 18" block with knee bent at 90 degrees, the other leg down on the floor straight out with foot propped up on side. Knee is pointing straight up towards ceiling on leg on floor, arms out to side palms up. Relax and hold position for allotted time.

Psoas Stretch (Rolls)

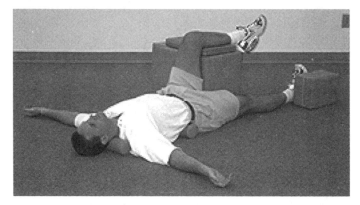

Lying on back with one leg on block with knee bent at 90 degrees, the other leg down on the floor straight out with foot propped up on side. Knee of down leg is pointing toward ceiling, a small roll under lower back and one under neck, arms out to side with palms up. Relax and hold position for allotted time.

Psoas Stretch (Progressive)

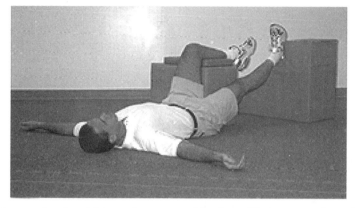

Lying on back with one leg up on block at 90 degrees, the other straight out propped up on outside of foot. The down leg is lowered incrementally toward the floor 5 inches at a time and stays at each level 3-5 minutes. Every time leg is lowered, the low back should slightly arch then flatten. Do not ever use a roll under back for this exercise. Relax entire time, arms out to side with palms up.

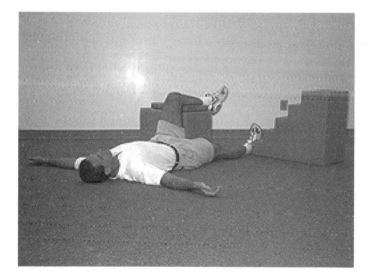

Push-ups (Walking Out)

Stand with feet hip width. Bend over at waist keeping legs straight, and walk hands out to push-up position. Separate hands wider than shoulders and bend elbows at 90 degrees with shoulder blades squeezed. Continue for the desired repetitions, then walk hands back toward feet and repeat.

Rolls (Settle)

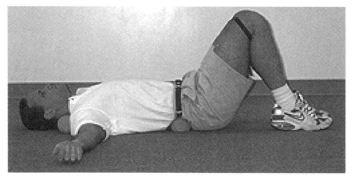

Lying on back with knees bent, feet hip width, place a roll under low back and neck. Settle and relax making sure head is on floor, knees resting out against strap. Place arms at side, palms up and breathe through diaphragm.

Rolls (Standing)

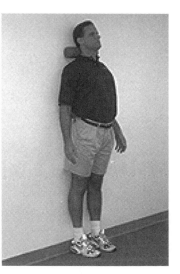

Stand with back against wall, feet hip width, stomach relaxed. Place roll behind lower back and neck while maintaining contact with wall at heel, buttocks, shoulders and back of head. Keep stomach relaxed entire time. You may feel this in calves and low back. Breathe.

Rooster Pose

Stand with palms of hands placed on upper glutes, feet straight and hip width. Keep arch in low back and bend at waist until arch in back begins to flatten. HOLD THERE. Press elbows together and bow back keeping weight on balls of feet. Keep quads tight and feel in hamstrings. Relax stomach.

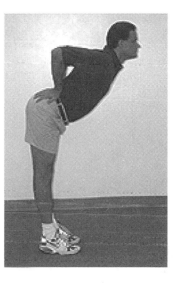

Rotator Cuff Sequence

Position 1: Standing with feet straight and hip with, make a slight fist with thumbs pointing to side. Keeping shoulder blades squeezed together, lift arms straight out to side slightly in front of body keeping thumbs pointing to floor. Do not shrug shoulders on way up and lower arms back in same direction. Repeat for allotted number of times. Relax stomach. Position 2: Lying on side with head propped on hand, slightly bend knees and place arm at side. Bend arm to 90 degrees and while keeping elbow at hip, rotate arm to floor until knuckles touch floor. Keeping wrist from bending, rotate arm back until knuckles point to ceiling not allowing body to rotate through motion. Repeat for allotted number of reps then switch sides. Relax stomach. Position 3: On back with knees bent, feet hip width and straight, place one arm at side with elbow bent to 90 degrees. Keeping elbow at side, rotate arm until back of hand touches floor keeping the right angle at elbow. Return arm to upright position and repeat for allotted amount of reps, then switch arms. Relax stomach and breathe. Position 4: On back with knees bent, feet hip width and straight, place arm straight out to side and bend elbow at 90 degrees with palm facing forward. Rotate arm until back of hand touches floor keeping right angle at elbow. return arm to upright position and repeat for allotted amount of times, then switch arms. Relax stomach and breathe.

Shin Burners (Static Floor)

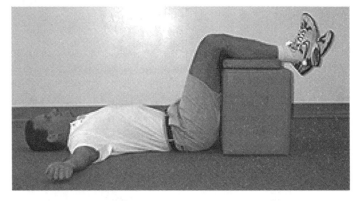

On back with knees bent at 90 degrees, on an 18" block. Rotate one ankle clockwise in full range of motion for allotted repetitions, then reverse direction. After both rotations, point and flex toes for allotted amount of reps, then switch to other ankle and repeat.

Shin Burners (Supine)

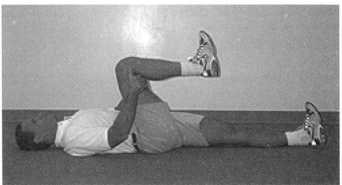

On back with one leg straight and the other bent and pulled back towards the same-side shoulder, rotate ankle clockwise in full range of motion for allotted repetitions, then reverse direction. After both rotations, point and flex toes for allotted amount of reps. Then switch to other ankle and repeat. Keep straight leg tight with toes pulled back during rotations of other ankle, keeping knee pointing to ceiling.

Shoulder Rotations (Gravity Drop)

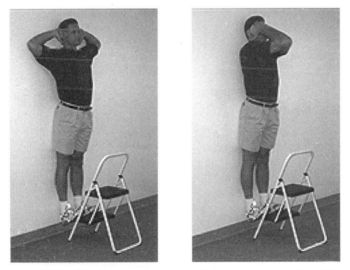

Stand on an Incline board (or step ladder) against wall with legs straight (do not bend knees), feet straight and hip width. Relax stomach and let body weight sink into heels. Position hands in golfer's grip and place knuckles on temples. Keeping knuckles on temples the whole time, bring elbows together. Then separate elbows by pulling arms back, squeezing shoulder blades together and bringing elbows to wall. Keep stomach relaxed.

Shoulder Rotations (Kneeling)

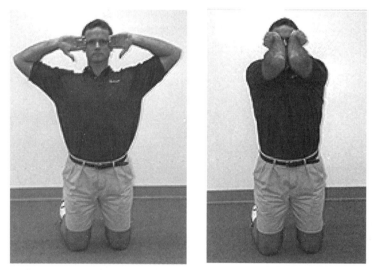

Kneeling with knees hip width apart, position hands in golfer's grip and place knuckles on temples. Keeping knuckles on temples the whole time, bring elbows together. Then separate elbows by pulling arms back, squeezing shoulder blades together. Keep stomach relaxed.

Shoulder Rotations (Sitting)

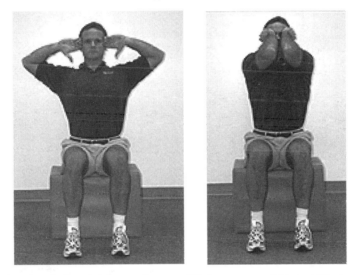

Sitting in chair with knees bent at 90 degrees and hip width apart, roll hips forward pushing stomach out to create arch in low back. Position hands in golfer's grip and place knuckles on temples. Keeping knuckles on temples the whole time, bring elbows together. Then separate elbows by pulling arms back, squeezing shoulder blades together and bringing elbows to wall. Keep stomach relaxed.

Shoulder Rotations (Standing)

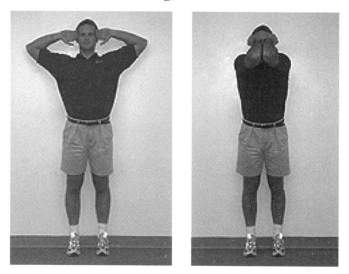

Standing with feet hip width apart and pointing straight ahead, position hands in golfer's grip and place knuckles on temples. Keeping knuckles on temples the whole time, bring elbows together. Then separate elbows by pulling arms back, squeezing shoulder blades together and bringing elbows to wall. Keep stomach relaxed.

Shoulder Rotations (Static Floor)

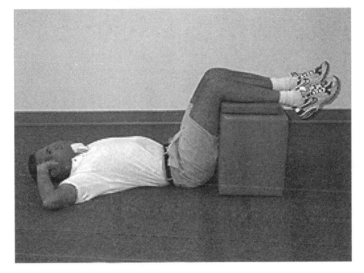

With legs propped up on 18" high block, knees bent at 90 degrees, position hands in golfer's grip and place knuckles on temples. Keeping knuckles on temples the whole time, bring elbows together. Then separate elbows by pulling arms back, squeezing shoulder blades together and bringing elbows to wall. Keep stomach relaxed.

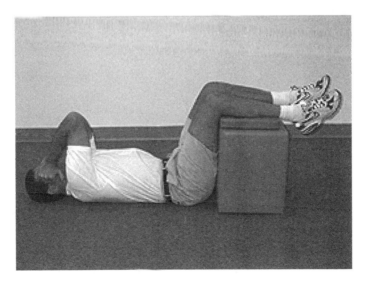

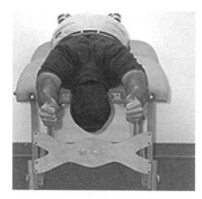

Shoulder Sequence

Lie on stomach with arms hanging over a counter top or edge of table, pigeon toe feet and let head relax down. Position 1: Point thumbs at each other, rotate thumbs to ceiling and raise arms over head keeping arms straight, then back down again. Repeat for allotted number of reps. Position 2: Raise and

lower arms at a 45 degree angle. Position 3: Raise and lower arm straight out to side at a 90 degree angle. Position 4: Bend elbows to 90 degrees with thumbs pointing at each other, elbows pointing to

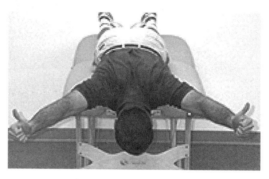

ceiling. Rotate thumbs away and from shoulder rotate arms up, thumbs to ceiling, without pulling elbows back. In all positions, relax buttocks and stomach.

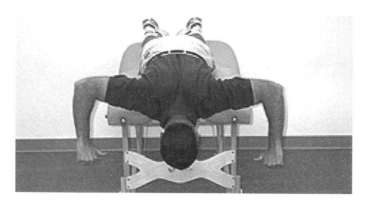

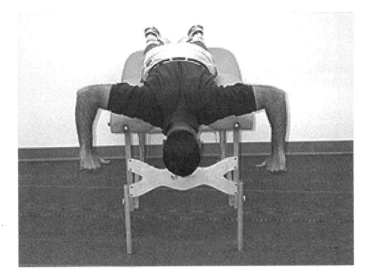

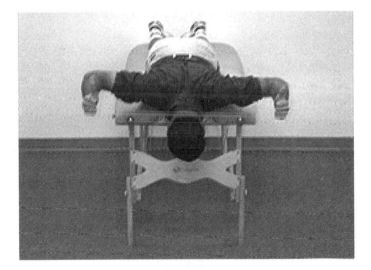

Sitting Knee Lifts (Pillow)

Sitting in chair with knees bent at 90 degrees and hip width apart, roll hips forward pushing stomach out to create arch in low back. Holding pillow between knees, lift knees up by leaving toes on the floor, then returning heels to floor. Focus on hip flexors lifting knees up and not calves pushing knees up. Keep arch in low back. Do not lean upper body back when lifting knees up, and relax stomach.

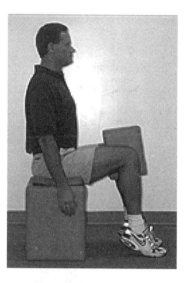

Sitting Knee Lifts (Strap)

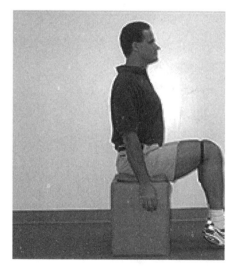

Sitting in chair with knees bent at 90 degrees and hip width apart, roll hips forward pushing stomach out to create arch in low back. Holding out against strap at knees, lift knees up by leaving toes on the floor, then returning heels to floor. Focus on hip flexors lifting knees up and not calves pushing knees up. Keep arch in low back, do not lean upper body back when lifting knees up, and relax stomach.

Sitting Knee Lifts (Unilateral)

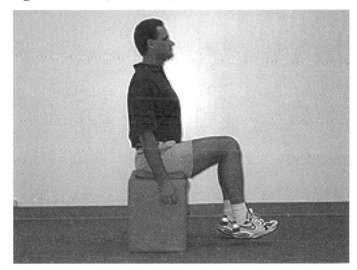

Sitting in chair with knees bent at 90 degrees and hip width apart, roll hips forward pushing stomach out to create arch in low back. Raise right heel while keeping toes on floor and lift left leg and foot off floor 3-4" keeping knee bent at 90 degrees. Slightly shift weight into the leg that is lifting, keeping arch in low back. Perform allotted amount of reps and then switch legs.

Sitting Knee Sequence

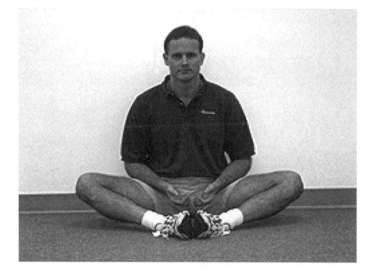

Position 1: Sitting on floor with back against wall, bend both knees and bring soles of feet together. Keeping shoulder and stomach muscles relaxed, let knees drop out to side and hold position for 1 minute. Position 2: From position 1, straighten one leg out in front with foot and knee pointing to ceiling. Tighten the quad muscle of the extended leg and pull the toes back. Press bent knee towards the floor using hip muscles. Keep shoulders and stomach relaxed and hold position for 1 minute. Switch legs and repeat. Position 3: From position 2, straighten both legs in front of body. Keeping knees and feet pointed towards the ceiling, tighten both quads and pull toes back. Keep upper body and stomach relaxed and hold for 1 minute. Position 4: Return body into position 1 with soles of feet placed together. Using muscles in the hip, press both knees to floor and hold for 1 minute. For every position the tailbone should be against wall or as close as you can get it. After each positional change, replace tailbone back against wall if it has slipped away.

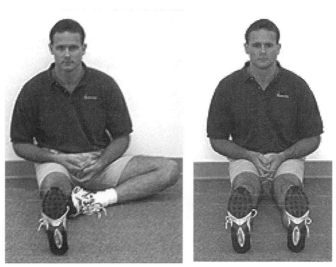

Position 2   Position 3

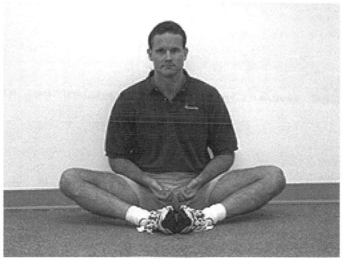

Position 4

Sitting Leg Lifts (Floor)

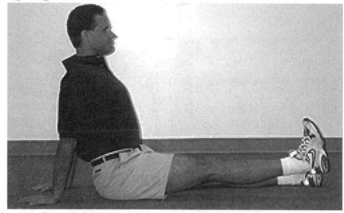

Sitting on floor with hands propped behind back, keep legs straight out and hip width. Pull toes back, tighten quads with knees pointing to ceiling, push stomach out and keep relaxed. Pull shoulder blades together without shrugging shoulders and lift one leg at a time up and down without losing arch in low back.

Sitting Leg Lifts (Wall)

Sitting against wall with tailbone as close to wall as possible, place back of hands on thighs, keeping legs straight out and hip width. Keeping tailbone against wall, pull toes back, tighten quads with knees pointing to ceiling, push stomach out and keep relaxed. Pull shoulder blades together without shrugging shoulders, and lift one leg at a time up and down without losing arch in low back.

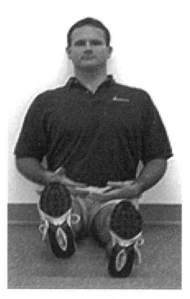

Sitting Leg Rotations

Sitting on floor with hands propped behind back, spread legs slightly wider than hip width. Tighten both quads, pull toes back and while maintaining arch in low back, rotate legs in and out without bending knees. Keep stomach relaxed out and do not shrug shoulders. Feel in hips.

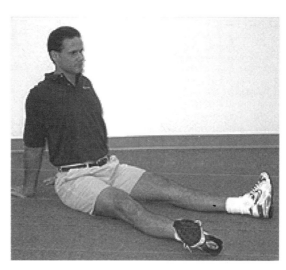

Sitting Side Stretch

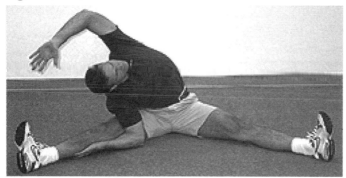

Sitting on floor with legs straight and spread apart, place right elbow inside of right leg with palm holding calf muscle. Keeping quads tight and toes pulled back (knees pointing to ceiling), arch low back by rolling hips forward, and lean towards right hip without lifting left buttocks off floor. Take left arm and reach overhead towards right foot keeping back arched. Hold for allotted time and switch sides, keeping stomach pushed out and breathe.

Sitting Torso Twist

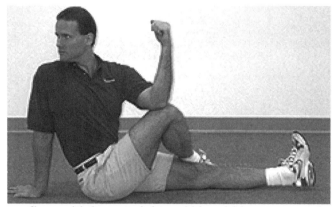

Sitting on floor with legs straight and hip width apart, prop hands behind back. Take left foot, bending leg, and place foot on outside of right knee (do not shift right leg inward). Place right elbow on left knee and sit up as tall as possible by arching low back. Tighten right quad with foot flexed back, pulling left shoulder back and twisting torso looking back over left shoulder. Do not push off right arm and keep stomach relaxed. Hold for allotted amount of time and switch sides.

Sitting Shrugs

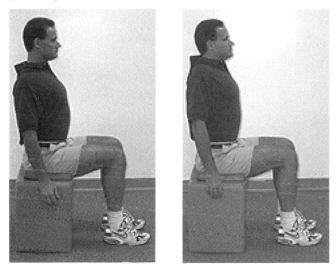

Sitting with knees bent at 90 degrees, place feet hip width and straight. Sitting up tall by rolling hips forward, creating arch in low back, pinch shoulder blades together and slowly raise them up towards ceiling and back down again. Keep shoulder blades pinched together the whole time and keep stomach relaxed and pushed out. Breathe!

Sobriety Glute Squeezes

Stand with one foot in front of the other, legs straight and balanced over both feet. Allow stomach and shoulders to relax and squeeze and release glutes without tightening quads or stomach. Perform allotted reps then switch feet.

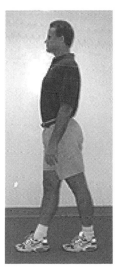

Squat

Hold on to waist-high support (sink, open door, etc.), with feet hip width and straight and close to support base. Allowing arms to straighten, arch back and sit down until knees are bent to 90 degrees holding back into extension and keeping knees directly over ankles. Keep shoulders and stomach relaxed, breathe and hold for allotted time. Feel in thighs and hip flexors.

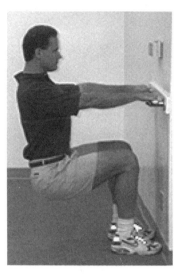

Squat to Stands

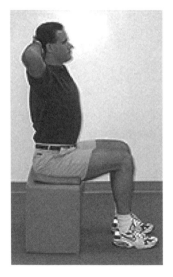

Sitting half way off chair, create arch in low back by rolling hips forward and pushing stomach out. Keeping knees at 90 degrees, place hands interlaced behind head and pull elbows back. Without leaning forward and losing arch in back, stand to full upright position using hips as much as possible. Return to sitting position by maintaining arch in low back and resisting forward leaning of torso. Repeat.

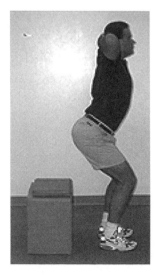

Standing Clock

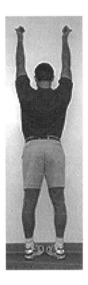

Standing facing wall with feet pigeon-toed, quads tight, extend arms straight overhead while keeping forehead on the wall. Make a fist and point your thumbs toward each other. Relax stomach and rotate arms (thumbs) away from each other at the shoulder joint. Shrug shoulders down to keep neck muscles relaxed. Hold position then repeat at 45 and 90 degree.

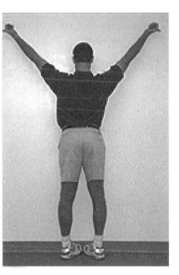

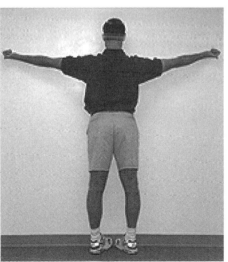

Standing Overhead Reach

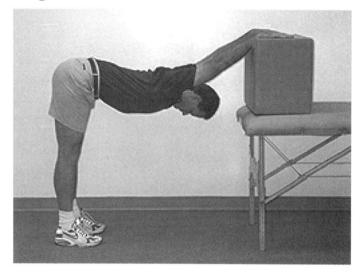

Place palms on waste-high counter with feet hip width apart and feet pointing straight ahead. Keeping hips directly over ankles, bend at waist, quads tight, arch low back allowing head and stomach to drop towards floor. Keep stomach relaxed and maintain weight on balls of feet. Feel in hamstrings and back.

Standing Shrugs

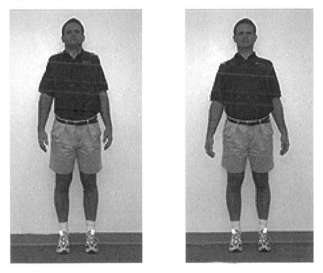

Standing against wall with feet straight and hip width, keep heels, butt, and shoulders against wall. While allowing stomach to relax, pull shoulder blades together and slowly slide them up towards ceiling and back down again, keeping shoulder blades pinched and against wall the whole time. Do for allotted repetitions.

Standing Splits

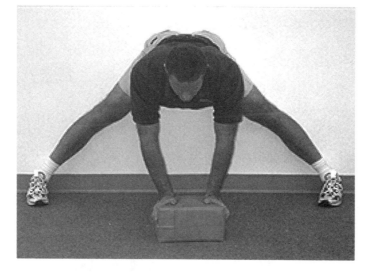

Standing with feet spread and pointing straight ahead, place heels and buttocks against wall. Tighten thighs and bend at waist keeping back as flat as possible and hold for 30 seconds. After allotted time, move hands to right foot. Hold for 30 seconds, keeping both glutes on wall and back as flat as possible. Then move hands to left foot maintaining same position and hold for 30 seconds. Then back to middle for another 30 seconds. Keep quads tight and breathe.

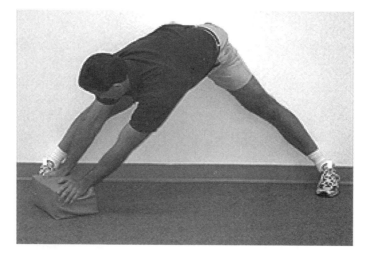

Static Floor

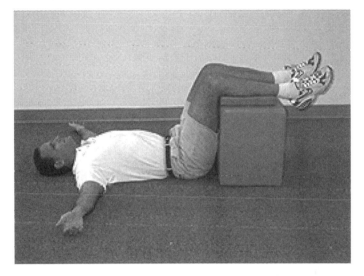

Lie on back with both legs on block and knees at 90 degrees. Keep arms out to side with palms up. Relax back into floor and breathe through diaphragm. Stay in position for allotted amount of time.

Step-Ups

Keeping feet hip width, place right foot on chair and step up onto chair by using right leg only. Keep body upright and straight with hips in extension. Step down with right foot first then switch legs. Can be done with arms at side, shoulders pulled back, or with hand interlaced on head with elbows pulled back.

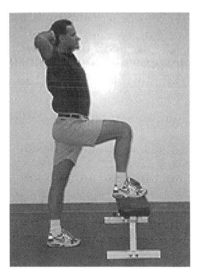

Straight Arm Rotations (Floor)

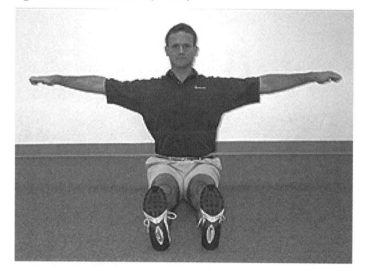

Sitting on floor with quads tight and toes pulled back, roll hips forward while pushing stomach out. With hands in golfer's grip position, raise arms from side keeping shoulder blades squeezed together without shrugging shoulders. Start rotations with palms facing floor, following thumbs forward over the top in approximately 6" circles. Then switch with palms facing ceiling and following thumbs forward over the top.

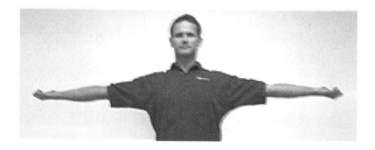

Straight Arm Rotations(Kneeling)

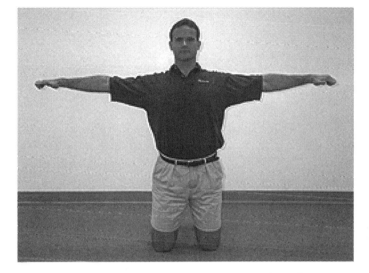

Kneel on floor with knees hip-width apart and STOMACH RE-LAXED. With hands in golfer's grip position, raise arms from side keeping shoulder blades squeezed together without shrugging shoulders. Start rotations with palms facing floor, following thumbs over top in approximately 6 " circles. Then switch with palms facing ceiling and follow thumbs backwards over the top.

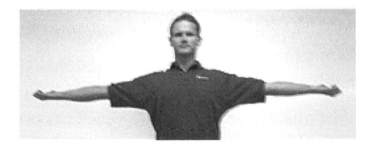

Straight Arm Rotations(Sitting)

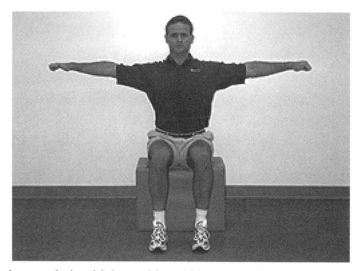

Sitting on chair with knees hip-width apart and bent at 90 degrees, roll hips forward and push stomach out. With hands in golfer's grip position, raise arms from side keeping shoulder blades squeezed together without shrugging shoulders. Start rotations with palms facing floor, following thumbs over top in approximately 6" circles. Then switch with palms facing ceiling and follow thumbs backwards over the top.

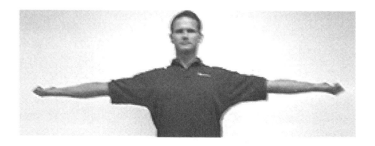

Straight Arm Rotations (Standing)

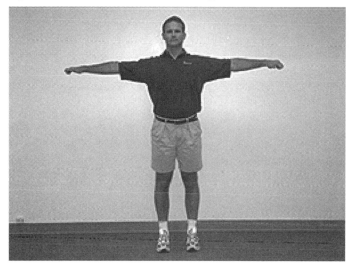

Stand with feet straight and hip-width apart looking straight ahead. With hands in golfer's grip position, raise arms from side keeping shoulder blades squeezed together and without shrugging shoulders. Start rotations with palms facing floor, following thumbs over top in approximately 6" circles. Then switch with palms facing ceiling and follow thumb backwards over the top.

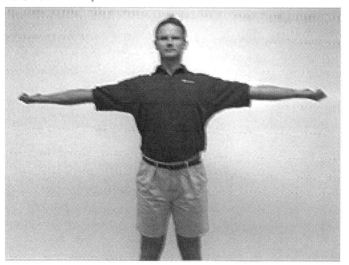

Striking Cobra

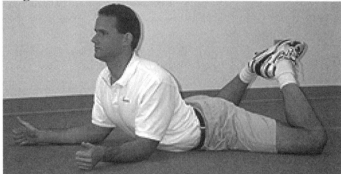

In prone position, prop elbows under shoulders and pull forearms apart while keeping hands on floor. Keeping shoulder blades squeezed together, separate legs, bend knees and press and release soles of feet flat together, keeping heels close to buttocks. Feel in glutes. RELAX STOMACH.

Striking Cobra (PBF)

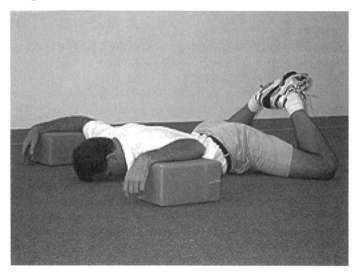

In Prone Blocked Floor position, separate legs, bend knees and press and release soles of feet flat together keeping heels close to buttocks. Feel in glutes. RELAX STOMACH.

TFL Stretch

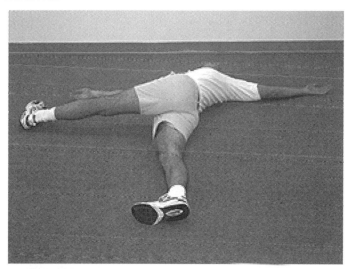

Start on back with legs straight out, knees and feet hip-width and pointing up to ceiling. Keep arms straight out from side with palms up. Tighten both quads, pull both feet back and raise one leg to 90 degrees to ceiling. Then rotate from the waist over to opposite side. Make sure that legs stay tight, feet flexed at the ankles. Look the opposite direction and keep stomach and upper torso RE-LAXED. BREATHE! Hold for allotted amount of time and then switch.

Toe Raises

Stand approximately 4" from door jam and hold on with both hands. Keeping body straight up and down, allow stomach to relax and back to arch. Position 1: Keeping feet hip width and straight, raise whole body as one unit up on toes towards ceiling without letting hips get closer to doorjamb, then back down to floor. Position 2: Keeping toes pointing out, repeat position 1. Position 3: Keeping feet pigeon toed, repeat position 1.

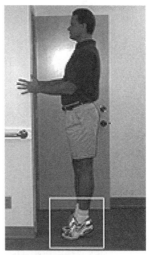

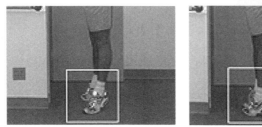

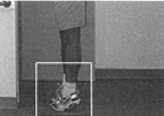

Triangle Position

Standing with right foot perpendicular to wall(heel on wall), rotate left foot so that it is perpendicular to the right foot and 3" off wall. Take a healthy step out with left foot keeping it 3" off wall. Place arms out to side with palms facing out, tighten quads and keeping both glutes and shoulders on wall rotate upper body from the waist towards the left foot. Slide down until right glute starts to come off wall, hold position and take right arm and stretch it over the top. Look up at right hand. BREATHE, and hold position for allotted time.

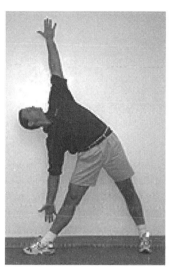

Turtle Pose

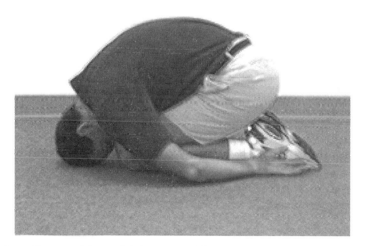

In kneeling position with knees and feet together, sit back on heels and allow upper body to drape forward. Allow head and shoulders to relax with arms at side, palms facing ceiling and let body settle into position.

Unilateral Knee Lift (Floor)

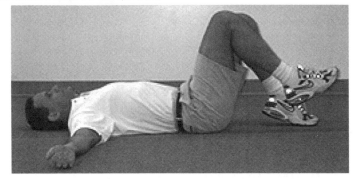

On back with knees bent and feet hip width, elevate one heel and leave toes on floor. Holding heel off floor, lift other knee towards shoulder 4-5" then return. Repeat for allotted amount of times; then switch. Keep shoulders and stomach relaxed while breathing through diaphragm. Alternate sets back and forth.

Unilateral Hamstring Stretch

Lying on back with one leg straight up on doorjamb and the other straight out on floor (foot blocked at side), tighten quad on elevated leg and pull toes back. Keep shoulders, stomach, and leg on floor relaxed and hold position for allotted amount of time; then switch. Make sure that buttocks stays on floor when leg is tightened.

Unilateral Hamstring Stretch (Progressive)

Lie on back with one leg straight up on doorjamb and the other straight out on 20" step, foot propped at side. Tighten quad on leg straight up, and pull toes back while relaxing the other leg. While keeping leg tight, progressively lower other leg down stairs in 5" levels every 4-5 minutes until leg is flat on floor. Relax shoulders and stomach and concentrate on breathing. Repeat other side.

Wall Groin Stretch

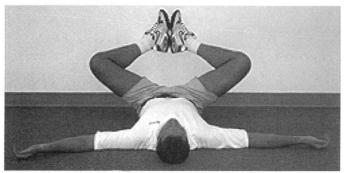

Lying on back perpendicular to wall, with buttocks as close to wall as possible, place soles of feet together bringing heels down wall as far as possible without separating feet. If buttocks comes off floor too much, then slide back off wall until you reach a more comfortable position. Place arms out to side and concentrate on breathing and relaxing. Feel stretch in groin. Hold position for allotted amount of time.

Wall Push

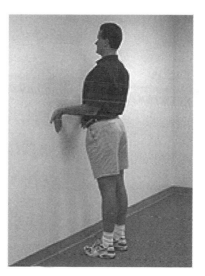

Stand Facing wall 6-8"away from wall with feet straight and hip-width. With arms at side, bend elbows at 90 degrees, palms facing ceiling, keeping elbows at side. Slowly lean into wall allowing hands to bend backwards and palms to be flat against wall. Hold position while shoulder blades squeeze together, keeping stomach relaxed and legs straight.

Wall Sit

With low back against wall, slowly walk feet away from wall. Keeping feet hip-width apart and straight ahead, slide down wall until knees are at 90 degree or just above. Keep weight on heels while pressing low back into wall and hold. Keep stomach and shoulders relaxed. Feel in thighs.

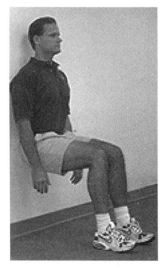

Wall Squeezes

Standing with feet straight and hip width, place heels against wall with buttocks and head against wall. Place arms at a 35 degree angle away from body, against wall so that the back of forearms and back of hands touch wall. Squeeze back of hands and forearms against wall so that shoulder blades squeeze together and then release. Do one set with head against wall and another with head hanging. Do the same thing with palms

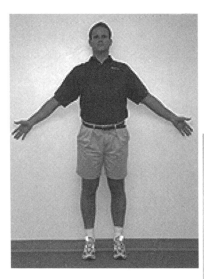

facing wall.

Wall Squeezes (Gravity Drop)

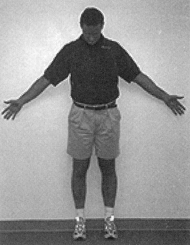

In Gravity Drop position, stand with feet straight and hip width, place heels almost against wall with buttocks and head against wall. Place arms at a 35 degree angle away from body, against wall so that the back of forearms and back of hands touch wall. Squeeze back of hands and forearms against wall so that shoulder blades

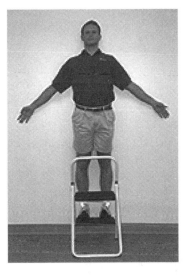

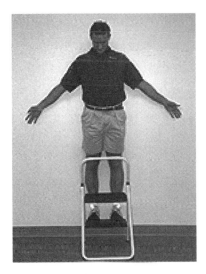

squeeze together and then release. Do one set with head against wall and another with head hanging. Do the same thing with palms facing wall.

Wall Twist

Place left foot slightly in front of the right, keeping feet parallel to wall, 1" away from wall. Place hands on wall, and while relaxing the whole upper body tighten both quads and twist left hip towards wall. Remain vertical and balanced on both feet while holding twist. Breathe.

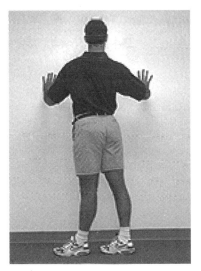

Symmetry
Enhanced Health
And Performance

Appendix Section

Richard R. Johnson
Patrick R. Mummy

Richard R. Johnson

Richard R. Johnson has enjoyed a multifaceted career as a writer, consultant, computer programmer, engineer, chemist, producer, musician, sales trainer and speaker. Perhaps his best attribute can be summed up as enthusiastically restless. Mr. Johnson currently resides in Southern California and enjoys a very active lifestyle, including a large family and surfing as often as possible. He is currently working on several publishing projects including topics on patents, communication automation and entertainment. Most of his projects utilize interactive multimedia delivered on CD-ROM to assist with subject emphasis and concept delivery. Mr. Johnson can be reached through the Quantum Media, Inc. offices by fax: 630-759-4846

Patrick R. Mummy

Patrick R. Mummy is the president of Symmetry. He earned a baseball scholarship to San Diego State University. His career rewarded him with numerous awards: The Western Athletic Conference Scholar Athlete Award, All District NCAA Baseball Team, NCAA Division One Baseball Scholarship, the Taylor and Edwards Memorial Athletic Scholarship, and Most Valuable Player for the Aztecs Baseball Team. His professional journey began through his formal education in Sports Medicine, which exposed him to the principles of biomechanics, kinesiology, exercise physiology, and anatomy. Through his experience, Patrick became aware of injury prevention and performance enhancement. He has performed on-site presentations at many leading corporations in the San Diego area, such as Qualcomm, Gen Probe, Sony, the FBI, Hyatt Regency, Mission Federal, Hallmark, and SDGE. He has sponsored many community events such as the Cancer Society's Jim Laslovic Golf Tournament, the Leukemia Society Marathon, and the Easter Seals Annual Wine and Cheese Event. He was recently featured on KUSI Channel 9 News.

Tom Palmer Creative Multimedia Producer

Tom Palmer is one very busy creative art director. He has developed a series of internet travel guides and a CD-ROM regarding the Year 2000 Computer Crisis. He has also developed a new interface design for the Oscar Mayer website and concepts for the KraftFoods Interactive Kitchen website for J. Walter Thompson advertising in Chicago. Tom has provided art direction and interactive programming on CD-ROM projects for Quantum Media in La Jolla and our Del Mar facility. For you pet lovers out there, Tom developed the Heinz Petfood Products internet site.

Pat Saylor

Pat Saylor has been an educator at Southern California community colleges for the past twenty-two years. She currently teaches English courses at Long Beach City College and is editing her own book: *Opportunities for Success in English Composition.*

Contact Information

Symmetry The Pain Relief Clinic
1104 Camino Del Mar, Ste. 101
Del Mar, CA 92014
619-794-0682

Quantum Media
1340 Enterprise Drive,
Romeoville, IL 60446
630-759-4666

README

This book and CD-ROM combination is meant to be used as a "Tag Team Approach," and we expect that most of our users will go back and forth from the book to the CD-ROM as needed. I strongly recommend that you cover as much information as you can from both sources to make your searches as fast and efficient as possible.

What's on the CD-ROM?

The CD-ROM includes the following:

1. The interactive program, "Symmetry."
2. System software programs that help run audio and video.

You can learn a great deal of information just from this book alone, but if you have access to a multimedia computer, there just may be no stopping you. Before you rush off there are some things you should know to make your time the most effective. If you spend a little time assembling and understanding some of the basic techniques, it will save you a great deal of time down the road. It helps to have a reasonable and realistic understanding of the equipment included with your computer set up. But this book and CD-ROM program are here to change all that, and bring as much information as is legally allowed to your fingertips.

Technology has brought us capable computers and decent Internet connections. One of the main things that we consider is the computer and other tools that you might use to help with the exercies. If experience has taught me anything, it's that most people who have a genuine desire, but lack experience with computers, will soon lose interest, become frustrated and give up.

Frustration with technology is perfectly understandable, and makes absolute sense to me, because if I did not make my living via computer technology, I would have thrown my computer in the trash

many years ago. It isn't so much that the technology doesn't deliver—it's that quite often the hype exaggerates the capability and
speed of delivery. Our expectations greatly exceed the capabilities
hyped by computer, software and Internet providers. People are
told faster computers and modems deliver information more
quickly. But experience dictates that computers generally become
faster to run more demanding software, so in the end, speed and
efficiency are about the same with a few more features than the
prior versions.

But for those with realistic expectations and a little patience, comes
a pot of gold at the end of the rainbow. If you learn to harness this
technology, or if you already know what you're doing, then the
rewards can be almost limitless. That's the promise that this technology will deliver, but first you have to get real.

Those who understand how to harness the technology offered via
the Information Age will without question prosper in their given
fields. They will find that the once daunting, seemingly impossible task of mastering the computer will become a game which is
fun to play, reasonably challenging and always exciting. When
you master the art of computer information retrieval, you have
opened the door to a world so vast and limitless that boredom and
apathy may cease to exist in your life.

Since we are utilizing a new technology, we will discuss how to
become more efficient with your computer and your time schedule. As we are discussing, and in many cases introducing people
to a brand new technology, there is some groundwork to be laid,
and there must be a general understanding of how and why certain
things are done. We have taken into consideration the pains and
frustrations that many people feel regarding computers in general.
No doubt we have experienced almost every problem that someone could have with our program during the development phase.
We consider these issues because we are showing people how to
improve their own health using a computer as a tool. If you have
trouble working computers, or have misconceptions that might prevent you from completing your goal, then these areas must be

handled first.

This is a two-part program, and hopefully the combination will prove to be the most powerful health assistance tool available. The book portion of this program outlines much of the basic information you need for a clear understanding, and the CD-ROM portion walks you through step-by-step. Please don't skip through the process and assume you have a handle on the subject matter unless you are an expert on whatever topic we're presenting. Skipping over important background information will only cost you time and frustration in the end.

For almost twenty years, I have instructed people on the use of efficiency technologies and as technology allowed, computer instruction. The key point is that valuable information can be revealed to you almost instantly using a CD-ROM. But you need some basic understanding before you go running off.

Some people like to do things in a slow, methodic way. In fact, I know several people who choose hand tools over power tools when both tools are sitting next to each other on a workbench. Many people with computers containing wonderful word processing programs choose the typewriter as their writing tool. Far more than that choose pen and paper instead of a typewriter, when both are sitting on the same desk. I also know several programmers who choose to write their programs in longhand instead of using compiler programs.

We hope you enjoy our book and CD-ROM program as much as we did creating them. If you're wondering why we have created a dual version product, it's because we wanted to arm you with every possible advantage to quickly master Symmetry. Perhaps it is possible that you merely want to learn about the process , or maybe you'd like to teach others. Regardless, if you desire subject matter about the process of Postrual Therapy, you have come to the right place.

The program "Symmetry" is a multimedia program, which means

it has sound, visual graphics, video, interactive screens and even databases that you create yourself. It's actually quite complete: everything you need is there to help you. The one thing that's not part of the CD-ROM is the ability to take the information with you in a book format anywhere you go. That's why we also have the book. This way you have the best of both worlds: all the information and interactivity you want, and the ability to take most of the information with you anywhere you go, any time, like any other book.

There is one tool that we need to talk about, and that is your computer. One of the reasons that the program "Symmetry" became a book and a CD-ROM combination program, is because many of our clients had difficulty running the computer program all by itself. There are many reasons for this, but the main reason is a lack of understanding of computer capabilities. We apologize in advance to you computer experts out there who have no need for this information, but in the meantime, we have a genuine purpose here.

Let's Talk About Your Computer

Okay, let's start at the very beginning: do you have a computer? Well, if you don't you can certainly use our program on someone else's computer, or you can rent a computer at a computer rental location, or take one home with you. There are cafes springing up everywhere that have multimedia-capable computers and Internet connections—perfect. Either way, let's get back to the computer that you have, or intend to use.

Books are not multimedia—they are text and graphics only. Unfortunately, many computers are also text and graphics only. If you know and understand that your computer is multimedia-capable, then you have most of the information you need. But you do need to understand how to make a multimedia program work its best without any errors or system crashes.

The reason that computers crash when using multimedia software programs is that there is no single standard in the software industry. In reality, there are probably hundreds of standards, and that is the single biggest problem. Imagine how TV would work if every television program had a different electronic format. You would need one type of television to see one program, and another type of television to see a different program, and so on. That is exactly what has happened in the computer industry. You actually need different types of computers to run different types of software. Some programs need a Macintosh; some need Windows; others need NT. Then there are data systems, beta systems, CAD systems—the list goes on into the hundreds. In reality it's not as bad as all that, because consumer and general business computers come with system software that has the capability of running several different types of programs in several different program languages. But one of the main reasons computers crash is because of the conflicts that occur at the system level. One day soon, most information will be standardized for specific delivery on a specifically standardized computer operating system. This will force software developers and hardware developers to communicate and develop their programs and products in harmony so everything runs predictably. The Internet, for example, has chosen the HTML programming language as a standard for the World Wide Web. Prior to the HTML standard, there were countless programmers out there attempting to create "the worldwide communication standard programming language." It's a miracle that we got to a standard so quickly. Now let's see how fast the rest of the computer world can agree on a systems standard for basic business and home computer users.

If you have a fairly new Macintosh computer, then you're probably good to go right off the bat. However, the PC world is a little more complicated because there are so many possibilities within the PC world, and so many people providing the software and hardware solutions. Although the PC world is getting better every day, there are still millions of people out there who have trouble running multimedia programs on their multimedia computers. In most cases, there is one simple problem. OK, two simple problems. I admit it—you've caught me—really, just a few main problems!

Problem No. 1

Old computer. You might have an old computer that simply is not capable of running today's programs. Many of today's programs require more memory, a larger hard drive, faster processors, color screens and so on. Certainly this is not your fault, and you should not be blamed in any way for hanging onto reliable, older equipment. But you know how technology goes, and sometimes you have to go with advanced technology if you want the best results.

Problem No. 2

Not Enough RAM. Just two or three years ago, most computers came with 4-8 MB of RAM. This situation has changed greatly over the last 18 months, and most new computers come with 32 MB of RAM, just to start. That's the good news. The bad news is that if you have only 4-8 MB of RAM you're probably going to need to upgrade. But not to worry, there's more good news: RAM has become very inexpensive, and you can likely pick up 32 MB of RAM for around fifty dollars.

Problem No. 3

No Video or Sound Card. Most new, brand-name computers come ready to go with video and sound cards. If for some reason, you have acquired a computer without video or audio capability, you will need to upgrade in order to experience multimedia. Be assured that most computer programs require the use of a video or sound card to get the most out of them. Once again, video and sound cards are not very expensive, and can be quickly installed where you purchase them—usually within five or ten minutes.

Problem No. 4

Software Entanglements. One of the most common ailments a computer can face is conflicting software, and it happens quite easily. Computer users often look for solutions and quick fixes to situations that can be managed from their computer. There are utility programs of almost every variety to help users manage their data. There are also thousands of shareware programs that people can try free of charge, but these programs can quickly clutter a hard drive and confuse an operating system.

The problem is that there are so many software programs out there, many of them conflict. For example, there may be three different "paint" programs, or three different word processing programs. Many computers have several utilities that all do the same thing, and it is common for these competing programs to conflict with each other. So at some point, if you look in your program directory or in your settings files, or on your hard drive, and you see several programs used for similar purposes, you should start deleting some of them. You can also use conflict-catching software that will help you find out if some of your programs are conflicting with others, with the overall result of confusing your computer system.

If you're not sure how to optimize your computer so that it will run its best, it's a very good idea to call a computer service/repair company and get their opinion. Most likely, they will be able to tell you how to optimize your system right over the phone. It might be as simple as defragmenting your hard drive. I realize that many of you have never heard of the term "defragmenting" your hard drive. I do not mean to be technical here, and it's not entirely necessary that you understand the technical characteristics of your computer. But put your mind at ease, because most other questions or issues regarding the technical aspects of your computer are in the Help section when you press the start button with your mouse with Windows 95 and 98. Macintosh help is usually found within the computer program itself or you can always use the "Find" command within the file menu.

A Word to the Wise and a Wish List for Those Frustrated by Computers. I understand that just about every word uttered about technical issues regarding computers can sound completely foreign and overwhelming to many. I believe that there is one quick and permanent fix to help anyone overcome apprehension and fear when working with computers. Go computer shopping and get yourself a nice, reasonably priced, multimedia-capable computer with a ton of RAM in a large hard drive, with a good modem and good-looking monitor. In other words, treat yourself to a new computer that will get the job done for quite some time. As this book is being written, there are several computers that cost less than fifteen hundred dollars and are incredible. You can even get a laptop with everything you need built right in. Maybe you can borrow someone's computer, or rent one, or consider working with someone else who has the equipment you need.

Almost on a daily basis, I have a conversation with a client or associate regarding computer communications. Typically the issue is that we want to communicate with each other, or exchange software in some manner. Perhaps there's a file type that we have in common—for example, a similar word processing program or database. The main issue or problem that always arises is one of compatibility, and typically people don't keep up with the latest upgrades and versions. When people are working on their own computers, and in essence doing their own thing, that's fine, and technology upgrades really don't matter. But when you begin to exchange files, or go on a network that is worldwide in scope and always upgrading. Using the Internet, you have no choice but to keep up with the latest software versions, such as the browsers which require the latest system upgrades and so on. You can see where this is going; when you make the decision to communicate with the big wide world on the Internet, you must automatically make the decision to continually upgrade your software and hardware configurations so you can be ready for anything.

The speed of information delivery often classified as "bandwidth" is continually being upgraded to meet the demands being placed on the Internet system. The more people, the more traffic, and that means greater demands on hardware and software all the way around. People in the compression business are always trying to find ways of making files such as pictures, sound and movies smaller. The idea is that the smaller the file size, the faster it will travel to its final destination through the Internet. But along with these new compression ideas comes the need for improved and upgraded software to handle the challenge. So the bottom line is: if you choose to venture online with your computer, be ready to upgrade, or stagnate.

What's Your Time Worth?

You might be thinking, "For heaven's sake, what have I got myself into? Here I'm considering the notion of improving my health, and we're talking about new computers and upgrades. What's going on?"

Every now and then, a little practical advice can be quite worthwhile, and this seems like the perfect place. Having spent most of my professional career accessing computer technologies to save time and money, I have learned some very valuable lessons. Mostly what I've learned is what I like and don't like regarding work and mundane tasks. I realized that I had choices about how I spent my time and how much time to relegate to a task. If the task was for enjoyment purposes itself, then time was not a factor. But if the task was to be completed as quickly as possible and time was money, then I always opted for the more efficient means to the end. I learned from my father and how he ran his business: if a new technology saved more time than it cost, you got it and mastered it. He was one of the first who went from carbon paper to a copy machine; from a hand ledger to a computerized accounting system; from letters to fax machines, and from print shops to desktop publishing. All the while, his business grew every year and he maintained a comfortable lifestyle with reasonable vacation time and free weekends. The lesson is simple, but often a hard pill to swallow: sometimes you have to make the move to a new technology to get the type of rewards in a time frame that only a new technology can deliver.

Note: If you recognize that a new technology is worthwhile but a little out of your reach, you can always rent or borrow from someone who has the latest technology on hand. Because after all, they may have the hardware, but what good is that without the coolest

software to go along with it? So you can bring the software, someone else has the hardware—no problem!

Treat Yourself — You're Worth It

There is nothing wrong with older technology, unless you want to
use it for something new. There's nothing more frustrating than
trying to get an old piece of equipment to perform a task beyond its
capabilities. The problem is, there are a lot of people out there
selling peripheral devices that are supposed to upgrade, but often
degrade the equipment they are supposed to improve. This situation is certainly one of the biggest time wasters ever. By the time
you research, shop for, and install the improvement, you probably
would have been able to offset the value of your time with the
purchase of new up-to-date equipment. Unless you are an equipment retrofit hobbyist, your best bet is to go with new, and not fool
around with time-wasting upgrades.

Have you ever actually sat down and tallied up what your time is
worth? You really should try it sometime, but you have to be realistic regarding your income or your income potential. First, consider how much money you make and write that down. Then how
much would it cost for someone else to do all of the mundane labor
that you perform around the house or office? The idea is to place a
value on everything you do, and your income as well, and that's
about what your time is worth. Next, try and assess how much
time you spend fiddling with your computer. There's a good chance
that you've given up altogether attempting certain tasks with your
computer. Maybe you had unrealistic expectations or maybe someone sold you a bill of goods, but either way, you're either wasting
time or not getting what you need and want out of your computer.

Most people who purchase computers, buy them with the hopes
that they will spend less time doing mundane tasks and achieve
greater efficiency. This is certainly a worthy goal and ideal, but
unfortunately, many people purchase computers that are incapable
of fulfilling their needs. Or many people buy computer parts and
pieces one at a time and things don't match up well. What ends up

happening is that they spend hundreds of hours spinning their wheels on a system that they don't understand, and frustration sets in. I see this and hear about this almost every day. Comparatively, the fix is easy and fast: purchase a computer which is well-suited to your desires and then run through the tutorials and manual word for word, page by page. Before you know it, you'll become an expert with your computer and find yourself doing things and saving time like never before. I know this first-hand because I have more spare time than almost anyone I know who does not utilize this incredible technology.

Why do we mention this? It's because we are offering a program designed for efficiency, utilizing every technological means possible and available to the everyday person. That pretty well sums up what computers and computer programs are supposed to. So, if we are offering a solution presented using concepts of efficiency, then we should talk about creating a path to greater efficiency for our software users. Basically, we want you to have more time to do the things you really want to do and spend less time doing the necessary evils. I am well aware of the demons that live inside many computers that caused their owners hour after hour trying to figure out what's wrong with their computer and why it won't work the way it's supposed to.

README

This is essentially the exact word-for-word README that you will find on the CD-ROM. The reason we put the ReadMe in the book is because most people won't read a README on disc. Regardless of how educated a software user is, most fail miserably regarding software instruction. The odd thing is that most computers and software come with at least a minimal amount of instruction to get you started. I have suggested that the CIA should transfer their most sensitive and secretive documentation via the README's that accompany most software, because most computer users are fatally allergic to README files. However, in a book format—not on disc—most people actually glance through a README, at the very least.

SYMMETRY README FILE

SYMMETRY - README - FOR WINDOWS & MAC

Thank you for buying "SYMMETRY." Before you use the program, take a few minutes to look through this readme file. It will help you to understand how SYMMETRY is organized and how to solve any problems that you may encounter.

FIRST STEPS

Go to your "My Computer" folder and open the CD-ROM folder called "SYMMETRY." This is where all of the folders and files reside for the CD-ROM program. There are two introduction programs for the CD-ROM called "Intro." One of them is for Mac users and the other is for PC users.

Step 1. Copy the folder that this "readme" is in onto your desktop. You don't have to do this, but it will make the program run a little faster if you do. Or use the Installer. There is no Installer for the Mac version.

Step 2. Double click on the "Intro" for Macs, or "Intro.exe," for Windows. We have included two different versions. You should hear sound and see an intro movie right away.

If you're unsure about any of these steps, you should refer to your manual, or in Windows 95, you can go to the Help section.

MAIN OBJECTIVE

The optimal use of this program is to master the concepts and techniques in SYMMETRY using the programs as it was designed with video, audio. Since we know there is no such thing as a standard computer configuration, we've designed the program so most computer users can utilize it, even if their computer setup is less than optimal.

Depending on your computer type, RAM, and supportive software, here are the basic strategies:

"Plan A" is to be able to experience video and sound.
If "Plan A" won't exactly work out, one of the following plans should.

"Plan B" is to run the program with sound, with no video.

"Plan C" is to run the program without sound or video, and do the best you can reading the information as it comes along.

Quick Overview Checklist:

1. Is your computer set up with new versions of "QuickTime" and "Sound Manager"? Well-tested versions of both are included on this disc.

2. Do you have enough RAM to operate the CD-ROM Program?

The rest of this file contains the following information:

I. Minimum System Requirements

II. More about the program

III. Instructions

IV. Known Errors and Workarounds

V. General Troubleshooting Tips

VI. More About Quantum Media

VII. Regarding Technical Support

VIII. License/Warranty/Disclaimer Information

PC MINIMUM SYSTEM REQUIREMENTS
IBM-PC compatible 486/66 MHz processor (or better)
8MB or more of RAM
Windows 3.1 (or greater)
DOS 5.0 (or greater)
1MB Super VGA card with VLB
Double-speed CD-ROM drive
16-bit sound card
MCI CD audio and MCI WAV audio support

QuickTime for Windows, version 2.0.3.
(You can install QuickTime from the CD-ROM if you don't already have it on your system.)

Macintosh MINIMUM SYSTEM REQUIREMENTS
68040 33MHz processor or better
8MB of RAM – **The more RAM the better...**
Double-speed CD-ROM drive
System 7.1.2 or greater
Mouse
QuickTime, version 2.0. (2.5 preferred)

MORE ABOUT SYMMETRY

SYMMETRY is a dynamic and informative CD-ROM title designed for all levels of computer users. The main purpose of the SYMMETRY CD-ROM is to provide information to assist with the often difficult and time-consuming process of improving personal health. This CD-ROM was designed with value in mind, and was created to provide information that one might learn at a seminar on the subject of Postrual Therapy. If one were to hire a professional to provide the same service, the costs could run from hundreds to even thousands of dollars. When a person wants to improve health, balance, energy and relieve pain, we believe that this program is the fastest and most economical means to that end.

NAVIGATION

At any time, you may navigate to other areas of the program by positioning the cursor on, and holding the mouse button down, on various click-able items on the screen. The program was designed to be intuitive and easy to follow. However, it is recommended that first-time users preview the entire program to get a clear understanding of its content and variety.

There are a few key commands that automatically navigate to certain areas:

TAB Key: Will restart the program.

"R" Key: Takes you to the Remote Control

UPPER 1, 2 and 3 Keys: Will change sound volume.
The operation of these keys can vary slightly from
system to system, and in some cases the 2 Key will
not change the sound levels.

We recommend that the first time you try the program, just surf through the entire CD. This way you can experience the full impact of the CD program.

INSTRUCTIONS
There are a few different ways you can operate this program:

A. Run it directly off the CD-ROM

B. Drag (copy) the "Mac" or "Win" folder onto your desktop depending on which system you have—Macintosh or Windows.

C. Double click on the "Start1.exe" or " Start2.exe" icon for Windows, or "Start" for Mac users.

D. Go through the introductory parts of the program so you'll have better results.

Windows 3.1

1. Insert the CD-ROM into the drive. Drag/Copy the"Win" file onto your desktop or click on the Installer.

2. Follow the ReadMe instructions on the screen.

3. Double-click on the "Win31.exe" program icon to play the CD.

Windows 95 or 98

1. Insert the CD-ROM into the drive. Drag/Copy the "Win" file onto your desktop or click on the installer.

2. Follow the ReadMe instructions on the screen.

3. Double-click on the "Start1 or Start2.exe" program icon to play the CD.

IV. KNOWN ERRORS AND WORKAROUNDS

Problem: In Windows 95, you may experience problems with distorted sound.

Solution: Obtain and install the latest drivers from your sound card manufacturer.

Problem: Your video and or sounds aren't working right.

Solution: Turn off ram doublers and/or virtual memory.

V. GENERAL TROUBLESHOOTING TIPS
If you want a favorable multimedia experience, make sure your computer is multimedia capable and up-to-date. RAM is the key, and most computers should have 32 Meg or more to successfully

operate today's multimedia programs. RAM solves most computer problems. Next, make sure you have workable versions of QuickTime from Apple. It is included on this CD for Mac and Windows.

Memory Issues For Windows

The more programs you have running in Windows at one time, the less memory is available for our program to use. This may result in an insufficient memory error message. To check which applications are currently running, press (CTRL+ESC) to open your task list. Close any unnecessary applications, and then rerun our program.

Disable any wallpaper you may have open in the background.

Make sure that you allocate a permanent swap file that is 7-10 megabytes in size. You may be losing out on accessible memory or performance if you have either a larger or smaller swap file. (For more information about swap files, refer to your Microsoft Windows documentation.) Windows 95 users should allow Windows 95 to control the size of the swap file instead of setting it manually.

If you're using SMARTDRV.EXE, add /X and /U to the command line to disable caching features that may interfere with smooth CD-ROM performance.

Sound
If you experience problems with the CD, we recommend that you try the following:

A. Try a music CD to check your audio card and software.

B. Check your cable connections.

C. Diagnose all applicable extensions and control panels.

D. Test your video card, if you're running Windows.

E. Disable RAM Doubling software, virtual memory or similar.

More Sound Issues

Make sure that you've installed and properly set up the most current drivers for your sound card. If you experience problems with distorted sound in Windows 95, obtain and install the latest drivers from your sound card manufacturer.

Make sure that your DMA, IRQ, and Port Address settings in Windows match the settings on your sound and video cards.

If you don't hear any sound when running the program, make sure that the mixer control for your sound card is turned up to an appropriate level. You should also make sure that your speakers are correctly plugged into the sound card.

DISCLAIMER

Quantum Media does not warrant or promise that the information herein will work with any or all computer systems.

Quantum Media does not assume any liability, either incidental or consequential, for the use of the information herein, including any and all damage to or lost use of computer hardware or software products, loss of warranties, or lost data by the customer or any third party. No oral or written information or advice given by Quantum Media, its employees, distributors, dealer or agents shall change the restriction of liability or create any new warranties. In no case shall Quantum Media's liability exceed the purchase price of the Quantum Media software product.

CD-ROM Handling

CD-ROM's are durable, but not indestructible. If you encounter problems, check for scratches on both sides of the disc. Scratches can make a disc useless, especially if any of the silver coating is chipped. Scratches can also cause read failures.

To clean your disc, wipe the shiny side with a soft, dry, lint-free cloth. Don't wipe around the disk (like you would a record). Rather, wipe from the center out to the edge. Repeat until the entire disc is clean.

Extra Mac Issues

Disable Unnecessary Extensions

Load only the extensions that are necessary to run the CD.

1. Hold down the space bar while the machine is booting up. This will open up the Extensions Manager panel.

2. Click on Sets.

3. Select All Off.

4. Select Custom.

5. Enable only the following extensions in the list for Macs:

a. Apple CD

b. QuickTime

c. Sound Manager

d. Foreign File Access

6. Save your extension set as "Symmetry".

By saving the set, you will be able to use it again the next time you want to run this configuration. The set name will appear in the Sets list. This new set becomes the default when you boot up. You must enable the other extensions in Extensions Manager to restore your

normal settings.
Memory Issues for Macs

Fine tune the memory settings to improve performance.
Lower the RAM Cache Size:
1. Open the System Folder, then open Control Panels.
2. Select Memory.
3. Set the Cache Size to 32k.

Disable Virtual Memory:
1. Open Control Panels.
2. Select Memory.
3. Make sure that Virtual Memory is set to Off.

Disable RAM Disk:
1. Open Control Panels.
2. Select Memory
3. Make sure that RAM Disk is set to Off.

Disable Modern Memory Manager (PowerMac users only):
1. Open Control Panels.
2. Select Memory
3. Make sure that Modern Memory Manager is set to Off.

If All Else Fails, Rebuild your Desktop.
1. Hold down the Command and Option keys while the system is booting up.
2. Choose OK, when asked if you want to rebuild the desktop file on the hard disk.

MORE ABOUT Quantum Media

Quantum Media produces industrial, consumer and educational Programs, and develops products under various publishing and distribution arrangements. The company consists of a group of professionals specializing in various aspects and production fields related to its titles. Quantum Media also creates interactive Hybrid music compact discs.

Quantum Media has created the STAR System, a fully automated system to assist with customer service, sales or any information exchange need related to telephone communication. They have designed an interface which directly connects a computer to a telephone for computer-assisted audio communications.
Check Out: http://www.cdpublisher.com and go to "Products."

Quantum Media's main objective is to provide helpful software that immediately supports and enhances practical day-to-day living and business pursuits. Our secondary goal is to design software that is automatically easy, and ready to use for anyone without need of manuals or frustrating technical requirements and support.

Our Web site is located at: http://www.cdpublisher.com

If you want to contact us via regular mail, write to us at:

Quantum Media
1340 Enterprise Drive
Romeoville, IL 60446

Regarding TECHNICAL SUPPORT
Our programs do not require any computer expertise to run smoothly and predictably. All operations are intuitive key strokes or mouse clicks accompanied by on-screen navigational instructions. To pause, click on "pause." There are forward and backward buttons, and so on. But we recognize that there will be something that has been overlooked for some computer users. The latest information and communication directions can be found at:
http://www.cdpublisher.com — click on "support"

LICENSE/WARRANTY/DISCLAIMER INFORMATION

The materials on this disc are copyrighted. Copying (except for personal archives), modifying or transferring the material is prohibited. hibited and in violation of the copyright law. All trademarks and copyrights are of their respective companies and/or owners. Limited Warranty: Quantum Media warrants that the CD-ROM is free of manufacturing defects for a period of 90 days from the date of receipt. Any implied warranties are limited to 90 days. Some states or territories do not allow limitations on duration or implied warranty, so the above information may not apply to you. Quantum Media's entire liability and your exclusive remedy, at our option, is replacement of defective product. This limited warranty is void if product failure is due to accident, abuse, or misapplication.

No other warranties: Quantum Media disclaims all other warranties, either expressed or implied. Quantum Media in no event shall be liable for any consequential damage whatsoever. This agreement is covered by state, territory and local laws.